Update Gastroenterology 2001

Recent Advances in Gastrointestinal Oncology

John Libbey Eurotext
127, avenue de la République
92120 Montrouge
Tél. : 33 (0) 1 46 73 06 60
e-mail : contact@john-libbey-eurotext.fr
http://www.john-libbey-eurotext.fr

John Libbey and Company Ltd
Collier House,
163-169 Brompton Road, Knightsbridge
London SW3 1 PY, England
Tel. : 44 (0) 20 75 81 24 49

CIC Edizioni Internazionali
Corso Trieste 42
00198 Roma, Italia
Tel. : 39 06 841 26 73

© John Libbey Eurotext, 2001
ISBN : 2-7420-0382-7

Il est interdit de reproduire intégralement ou partiellement le présent ouvrage - loi du 11 mars 1957 - sans autorisation de l'éditeur ou du Centre Français du Copyright, 6 *bis*, rue Gabriel-Laumain, 75010 Paris.

Update Gastroenterology 2001

Recent Advances in Gastrointestinal Oncology

Edited by
G.N.J. Tytgat, L. Lundell

Postgraduate Course 2001
Amsterdam, October 7

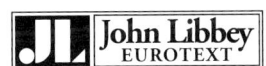

The publication of this book was made possible
thanks to the support from the Takeda Laboratories.

Contents

Foreword
G.N.J. Tytgat, L. Lundell 1

I – Management of GI Lesions with Malignant Potential

Barrett's esophagus and the role of complete acid control
D.O. Castell 5

Gastric atrophy and metaplasia: does *Helicobacter pylori* eradication suffice?
M.F. Dixon 11

Primary sclerosing cholangitis: prevention and/or specific therapy
S. Wagner, P.N. Meier, M.P. Manns 19

Dysplasia in ulcerative colitis: management principles
J.D. Waye 29

II – Novel Techniques for GI Tumour Removal

Mucosectomy: new therapeutic strategy in case of high grade intraepithelial neoplasia and early cancer of the upper GI-tract
C. Ell 39

Transgastric endoscopic approaches
H. Lönnroth 45

Transanal endoscopic microsurgery in the treatment of rectal tumors
E. Lezoche, M. Guerrieri 51

III – Ultrasound Guided Endoscopic Procedures

Endoscopic ultrasound guided fine needle aspiration. A critical appraisal
P. Vilmann, J. Thorbøll 63

EUS-guided celiac plexus neurolysis
P. Fockens 77

Cyst drainage procedures
T. Ponchon 81

IV – Endoscopic Procedures for Palliation

Treatment of malignant colonic stenosis with self-expandable metallic stents
R.A. Kozarek 93

Management of gastrointestinal lesions with malignant potential endoscopic techniques for palliation: laser techniques
Hugh Barr 101

List of contributors

Barr H., Cranfield Postgraduate Medical School in Gloucestershire, Gloucestershire Royal Hospital, Gloucester GL1 3NN, United Kingdom.

Castell D.O., Department of Medicine, Graduate Hospital, 1800 Lombard Street, Suite 501 Pepper Pavilion, Philadelphia, Pennsylvania, USA.

Dixon M.F., Academic Unit of Pathology, University of Leeds, Leeds LS2 9JT, United Kingdom.

Ell C., Department of Medicine II, HSK Wiesbaden, Germany.

Fockens P., Department of Gastroenterology, Academic Medical Center, University of Amsterdam, PO Box 22700, 1100 DE Amsterdam, Netherlands.

Guerrieri M., Clinica di Chirurgia Generale, Ospedale Umberto I, University of Ancona, Ancona, Italy.

Kozarek R.A., Virginia Mason Medical Center, 1100 Ninth Avenue, Seattle, WA 98101, USA.

Lezoche E., II Clinica Chirurgica, Policlinico Umberto I, "La Sapienza" University, Roma, Italy.

Lönnroth H., Sahlgrenska University Hospital, Göteborg, Sweden.

Manns M.P., Department of Gastroenterology and Hepatology, Medizinische Hochschule Hannover, D. 30623 Hannover, Germany.

Meier P.N., Department of Gastroenterology and Hepatology, Medizinische Hochschule Hannover, D. 30623 Hannover, Germany.

Ponchon T., Service d'Hépato-Gastroentérologie, Hôpital Édouard-Herriot, 5, place d'Arsonval, 69437 Lyon Cedex 03.

Thorbøll J., Department of Surgical Gastroenterology, Gentofte University Hospital, 2900 Hellerup, Denmark.

Vilmann P., Department of Surgical Gastroenterology, Gentofte University Hospital, 2900 Hellerup, Denmark.

Wagner S., Department of Gastroenterology and Hepatology, Medizinische Hochschule Hannover, D. 30623 Hannover, Germany.

Waye J.D., GI Endoscopy Unit, Mount Sinai Hospital, and GI Endoscopy Unit, Lenox Hill Hospital, New York 10021, USA.

Foreword

Pr Lundell and myself welcome you on behalf of the EAGE council to the traditional Postgraduate Course 2001. This postgraduate course is one of the many European educational activities of the EAGE. EAGE means EDUCATION of all aspects of gastro-entero-hepato-pancreatology.

The four main topics of this year's postgraduate course relate to digestive cancer: a) the management of GI lesions with malignant potential (Barrett's esophagus, atrophic gastritis with intestinal metaplasia, primary sclerosing cholangitis and colonic dysplasia); b) novel techniques for GI tumor removal (mucosal resection, transgastric resection, full thickness endoscopic resection), c) ultrasound guided procedures (fine needle aspiration, celiac plexus neurolysis); d) endoscopic palliative procedures (stenting, laser, etc.).

A galaxy of world re-known experts will cover these various topics which truly reflect cutting-edge developments. Their scientific and educational qualities guarantee a teaching performance of highest standard.

As is traditionally done, Pr Galmiche and the John Libbey publishing house did again a remarkable job in producing a superb syllabus, which signifies a nice addition to the unique and growing EAGE-syllabi library. This magnificent achievement was only possible through an unlimited educational grant from Takeda France for which the EAGE is sincerely grateful.

The course organizers trust that all participants will value this 2001 EAGE postgraduate course as outstanding.

        Pr Dr. G.N.J. Tytgat   **Pr L. Lundell**

I

Management of Gastrointestinal Lesions with Malignant Potential

Barrett's esophagus and the role of complete acid control

Donald O. Castell

Department of Medicine Graduate Hospital, Philadelphia, Pennsylvania, USA

Barrett's esophagus is an entity which has been immersed in questions and controversy since its original description in 1950 [1]. Barrett suggested that this columnar-lined esophagus represented a congenital short esophagus with intrathoracic stomach [1]. Allison and Johnstone subsequently supported the congenital origin of this condition, but did postulate that in some instances the condition might be acquired [2]. Stronger support for an acquired etiology began to be voiced over the next decade. Hayward was a proponent of the upward migration of the junctional epithelium of the esophagus and stomach [3]. A major breakthrough in the understanding of the pathogenesis of Barrett's esophagus occurred with the landmark publication of Bremner *et al.* reporting their ability to re-epithelialize a denuded segment of the squamous mucosa with columnar mucus-secreting cells in dogs with surgically-created persistent gastroesophageal reflux and induced gastric hypersecretion [4]. These investigators used the term "creeping substitution" to suggest a migration of columnar epithelium upward to replace squamous epithelium destroyed by persistent gastroesophageal reflux.

It is now accepted that Barrett's esophagus is an acquired condition and is one of the complications of chronic gastroesophageal reflux. It is also much more likely to be present in patients with other complications of severe gastroesophageal reflux disease (GERD) (*i.e.* esophageal ulcer or stricture). In fact, the common association between Barrett's epithelium and distal esophageal ulcers has led to the use of the term "Barrett's ulcer" to describe this condition. Most authorities in this field now agree that a true Barrett's epithelium consists of a "specialized columnar epithelium" (SCE) that resembles intestinal mucosa, with a villiform surface containing both columnar and goblet cells and with underlying crypts reminiscent of the lining of the small intestine (*i.e.* intestinal metaplasia). This is in contrast to the gastric type epithelium originally described by Barrett. Thus, even in its primary definition, the question of what truly constitutes a Barrett's esophagus has been controversial and often confusing.

Although much has been learned about Barrett's esophagus since 1950, many unanswered questions remain. There is general agreement about its pathogenesis and the association between this condition and adenocarcinoma of the esophagus. The appropriate therapy for Barrett's esophagus, whether uncomplicated or with evidence, remains very controversial.

If it is accepted that intestinal metaplasia of the esophageal mucosa results from chronic injury secondary to acid gastroesophageal (GE) reflux, it would seem to follow, that appropriate therapy of Barrett's esophagus, once recognized, should attempt to eliminate any continuing esophageal acid exposure. Indeed, the usual standard of care in this disease includes the use of potent acid suppressing medications (or surgery) in an attempt to accomplish this goal. Such therapies have been well documented to result in resolution of the patient's reflux symptoms and healing of associated esophagitis. There is, however, at present neither evidence nor consensus that either of these therapeutic approaches results in regression of the metaplastic epithelium or elimination of the malignant potential in this disease.

The perennial discussion regarding **long-term treatment of GERD in general and Barrett's esophagus in particular has been concerned with the risks and benefits of medical *versus* surgical approaches**. Improvements in both over the past decade have made modifications in this argument appropriate. The techniques of anti-reflux surgery have evolved to the point where laparoscopic approaches are readily applied in these patients, although no long-term follow up of laparoscopic fundoplication in patients with Barrett's esophagus is yet available. One review of six larger reported surgical series with follow up from 48 to 78 months has indicated little evidence for regression of the metaplastic epithelium and the occasional appearance of adenocarcinoma [5]. A more recent publication with follow up over 100 months of 152 patients with Barrett's esophagus having antireflux surgery indicates a symptomatic failure rate of approximately 60%, with 15 patients developing evidence of dysplasia and four patients having adenocarcinoma seven years following surgery [6].

Improvements in acid suppressive therapy with the advent of proton pump inhibitors (PPIs) now offer the opportunity for chronic effective control of esophageal acid exposure with no evidence of adverse side effects to date. Similar to the surgical series, however, there is lack of definitive evidence of regression of the metaplastic epithelium in reports of 67 and 72 months of follow up [7, 8]. However, gastric and esophageal pH monitoring in these patients has indicated that many, if not most, have not achieved effective deacidification of the metaplastic epithelium.

The question of whether more complete acid control, and with what regimen, will result in historic regression of metaplastic epithelium in patients with Barrett's esophagus remains to be resolved. The usual clinical approach of adjusting the dose of acid suppressing medication to achieve symptom relief is hampered by the fact that patients with Barrett's esophagus have been demonstrated to have decreased sensitivity to esophageal acid exposure [9]. A seminal report using intragastric and intraesophageal pH monitoring in such patients after achieving symptom relief demonstrated that 80% continued to have abnormal esophageal acid exposure, particularly over night [10]. This observation has more recently been confirmed in a larger group of patients [11]. Therefore, I recommend the approach shown in *Table I*. All patients with Barrett's esophagus should receive

Table I. Suggested therapeutic approach to Barrett's esophagus

- Initial approach: PPI BID AC (twice daily before breakfast and dinner)
- One month: pH monitor (esophagus and stomach) *on therapy* and endoscopy with biopsies
- Adjust treatment to control acid exposure by repeat pH monitoring
    PPI once daily (AM or PM AC)
    PPI BID AC
    PPI BID AC + H_2RA HS
    PPI TID AC + H_2RA HS

initial therapy with a proton pump inhibitor given twice a day, before breakfast and dinner. This should achieve symptomatic remission and healing of the esophagitis in the majority of patients. Dual electrode (gastric and esophageal) prolonged ambulatory pH monitoring should then be performed *on therapy* to document the adequacy of acid control. If the patient remains symptomatic, esophagitis has failed to heal, or pH metry reveals continuing esophageal acid exposure, the addition of a bedtime dose of ranitidine (300 mg) should control this nocturnal acid breakthrough [12], likely to occur in 70-80% of these patients [13, 14]. An occasional patient may require augmenting this regimen with a TID (before meals) dose of PPI plus bedtime ranitidine.

Does continuing acid reflux, even in diminished amount, constitute a threat to the patient with Barrett's esophagus? The first suggestion that this might be true was provided by cell culture studies from esophageal biopsies of patients with Barrett's esophagus which showed that *in vitro* exposure to pulses of acid resulted in greater proliferation and less differentiation of the metaplastic epithelium than either continuous acid or neutral pH media [15]. A subsequent study by these same investigators provided the clinical link to the *in vitro* experiments. Using ambulatory pH monitoring on therapy with a proton pump inhibitor to establish the presence or absence of control of GE reflux, these investigators documented that patients with continuing abnormal GE reflux showed greater evidence of proliferative activity and less differentiation from their endoscopic biopsies than did patients with well-controlled GE reflux [16]. Thus, experimental evidence both at the basic and clinical level supports the need for ambulatory pH monitoring to establish adequacy of acid suppression therapy and to guide titration of medication dosing in these patients.

Does dose adjustment based on pH monitoring result in evidence of regression of the abnormal metaplastic epithelium in Barrett's esophagus patients? There are two recent clinical observations that would suggest an affirmative answer to this question. Our approach to patients with Barrett's esophagus has been to use pH monitoring to adjust therapy with PPIs or the combination of PPIs and night time H2 receptor antagonists to produce "total control" of GE reflux. In an on-going uncontrolled clinical trial of nine patients followed on this regimen for an average of 30 months, we have observed linear regression of the Barrett's mucosa in all nine and the presence of squamous islands in six [17]. A more convincing observation was recently published by Peters *et al.* [18] in a controlled study of 26 patients with Barrett's esophagus treated for symptom relief by ranitidine 150 mg bid compared to 27 patients randomly assigned to receive omeprazole, 40 mg bid. Ambulatory pH monitoring was used to establish complete control of GE reflux in the omeprazole treated patients. At the end of 24 months of endoscopic follow up, these authors have shown evidence of significant regression in the area of the Barrett's metaplasia with complete acid control produced by high dose omeprazole therapy compared to the ranitidine treated patients.

Over the past decade, there has been accumulating evidence that the use of ambulatory pH monitoring to document control of acid reflux is a helpful adjunct in the treatment of patients with Barrett's esophagus. Hopefully, the weight of this evidence will convince more clinicians and investigators to ensure that their patients do not have continuing esophageal acid exposure eliminated and further evidence will become available that this approach may actually lead to regression of the metaplastic epithelium and potentially decrease the risk of developing malignant changes.

References

1. Barrett NR. Chronic peptic ulcer of the oesophagus and "oesophagitis." *Br J Surg* 1950; 38: 175-9.
2. Allison PR, Johnstone AS. The oesophagus lined with gastric mucous membrane. *Thorax* 1953; 8: 87-93.
3. Hayward J. The lower end of the oesophagus. *Thorax* 1961; 16: 36-47.
4. Bremner CG, Lynch VP, Ellis FH, Jr. Barrett's esophagus: Congenital or acquired? An experimental study of esophageal mucosal regeneration in the dog. *Surgery* 1970; 68: 209-16.
5. Sampliner RE. New treatment for Barrett's esophagus. *Semin GI Dis* 1997; 8: 68-74.
6. Csendes A, *et al*. Long-term results of classic anti-reflux surgery in 152 patients with Barrett's esophagus. *Surgery* 1998; 123: 645-57.
7. Sharma P, Sampliner RE, Camargo E. Normalization of esophageal pH with high-dose proton pump inhibitor therapy does not result in regression of Barrett's esophagus. *Am J Gastroenterol* 1997; 92: 582-5.
8. Cooper BT, Neumann CS, Cox MA, Igbal TH. Continuous treatment with omeprazole 20 mg daily for up to six years in Barrett's oesophagus. *Aliment Pharmacol Ther* 1998; 12: 893-97.
9. Johnson DA, *et al.* Esophageal acid sensitivity in Barrett's esophagus. *J Clin Gastroenterol* 1987; 9: 23-7.
10. Katkza DA, Castell DO. Successful elimination of reflux symptoms does not ensure adequate control of acid reflux in Barrett's esophagus. *Am J Gastroenterol* 1994; 89: 989-91.
11. Ouatu-Lascar R, Triadafilopoulos G. Complete elimination of reflux symptoms does not guarantee normalization of intraesophageal acid reflux in patients with Barrett's esophagus. *Am J Gastroenterol* 1998; 93: 711-6.
12. Peghini PL, Katz PO, Castell DO. Ranitidine controls nocturnal gastric acid breakthrough on omeprazole: a controlled study in normal subjects. *Gastroenterology* 1998; 115: 1335-9.
13. Peghini PL, Katz PO, Bracy NA, Castell DO. Nocturnal recovery of gastric acid secretion with twice-daily dosing of proton pump inhibitors. *Am J Gastroenterol* 1989; 93: 763-7.
14. Katz PO, Anderson C, Khoury R, Castell DO. Gastroesophageal reflux associated with nocturnal gastric acid breakthrough on proton pump inhibitors. *Aliment Pharmacol Ther* 1998; 12: 231-4.
15. Fitzgerald RC, Omary MB, Triadafiliopoulas G. Dynamic effects of acid on Barrett's esophagus. *J Clin Invest* 1996; 98: 2120-8.
16. Ouatu-Lascar R, Fitzgerald RC, Triadafilopoulos G. Differentiation and proliferation in Barrett's esophagus and the effects of acid suppression. *Gastroenterology* 1999; 117: 327-35.
17. Srinivasan R, Katz PO, Ramakrishnan A, Katzka D, Vela MF, Castell DO. Maximal acid reflux control on Barrett's oesophagus: Feasible and effective. *Aliment Pharmacol Ther* 2001; 15: 519-24.

18. Peters F, Ganesh S, Kuipers EJ, Sluiter WJ, Klinkenberg-Knol EC, Lamers CB, Kleibeuker JH. Endoscopic regression of Barrett's oesophagus during omeprazole treatment; a randomised double blind study. *Gut* 1999; 45: 489.

Gastric atrophy and metaplasia: does *Helicobacter pylori* eradication suffice?

Michael F. Dixon

Academic Unit of Pathology, University of Leeds, UK

For over a quarter of a century it has been widely accepted that the majority of gastric cancers arise through a multi-step process starting with chronic gastritis and progressing through atrophy, intestinal metaplasia (IM) and dysplasia to invasive carcinoma [1]. Corpus atrophy results in hypochlorhydria, which favours carcinogen formation, while atrophic gastritis and metaplasia are hyperproliferative states that favour mutagenesis. Thus atrophy and metaplasia are generally held to be premalignant conditions, although the strength of the association is disputed. More recently, it has been established that infection with *Helicobacter pylori* is a major risk factor for gastric carcinogenesis and, in keeping with this, infection has been directly implicated in the development of atrophy and intestinal metaplasia [2-4]. This poses the question "Can eradication of *H. pylori* reverse these premalignant conditions and interrupt the atrophy-carcinoma sequence?" In order to answer the question, one first has to understand the biology and natural history of these conditions and then explore the possibilities for their reversal.

The nature of atrophy

Atrophy in the stomach is conventionally (and simply) defined as "loss of glands". Such loss may follow ulceration with destruction of the glandular layer, or, more frequently, results from a prolonged inflammatory process in which multiple glandular units separately undergo destruction. However, atrophy can also be thought of as "a loss of specialised *cells*". Under this broader definition, it is possible to include loss of parietal and chief (zymogenic) cells without glandular destruction. Such partial or "pre-atrophy" has been described in human autoimmune gastritis [5] and is frequently encountered in animal models of both autoimmune gastritis [6] and chronic *Helicobacter* infection [7]. In these latter situations, oxyntic cells are replaced within the intact glandular tubules by mucous neck cells (MNC). More interestingly, partial loss of parietal cells and replacement by MNC are a frequent, but largely unrecognised, finding in the inflamed corpus in *H. pylori* gastritis [8]. MNC were originally considered to be a transit cell population intermediate between stem cells and the fully differentiated parietal and chief cells. However, the repertoire of trefoil peptides and growth factors produced by MNC indicate that they are a distinct cell lineage, which shares the properties of other mucosally-protective cell lineages in the gastrointestinal (GI) tract [9]. Furthermore, it is apparent that proliferation of MNC explains the appearance of new glands formed in the wake of atrophy, so-called "pyloric metaplasia".

There are two principal routes to atrophy, one in which the stem cell compartment and/or glands are destroyed either by direct injury or as a consequence of the host inflammatory cell response, and the second when selective destruction of specialised epithelial cells occurs with preservation of stem cells. Both routes may apply in chronic *H. pylori* infection; on the one hand, bacterial toxins or, more likely, proteases released by activated polymorphs could destroy glandular epithelium and stem cells [10], while on the other autoantibodies are produced which react with epitopes on the proton-pump in parietal cells [11].

The nature of intestinal metaplasia

Metaplasia represents a non-neoplastic change in cellular phenotype that usually arises in response to a sustained adverse environment. The altered phenotype is either a consequence of somatic mutation in stem cells or of epigenetic events which produce divergent differentiation in progeny cells. The subsequent emergence of the altered phenotype as the dominant population is a result of selection pressures exerted by the changed microenvironment [12, 13]. The pattern of gene expression determining cell phenotype is under the control of a complex hierarchy of transcription factors of which *homeodomain* proteins are important members. These proteins are themselves regulated by *homeobox* genes whose expression is pivotal to cellular differentiation and organogenesis [14]. Thus the homeobox genes *Cdx-1* and *Cdx-2* are normally only expressed in the intestine but a corresponding transcription factor (CDX-1 protein) is present in IM in the stomach [15]. However whether such expression results from a mutation in stem cells or epigenetic changes has not been determined. Certainly a wide range of genetic changes including telomere reduction, microsatellite instability and mutations in p53, APC and k-*ras* have been described in IM even before the onset of dysplasia [16].

IM can be divided into three sub-types which are likely to differ in their histogenesis and relationship to carcinogenesis, namely type I (complete) which closely resembles small intestine, type II (incomplete – goblet cell metaplasia) and type III (incomplete – "colonic" type). Interestingly it is the latter type that harbours most genetic changes [17, 18] and the only IM phenotype that carries a higher risk for gastric cancer [19].

Is reversibility possible?

In any consideration of reversibility of atrophy, a distinction has to be made between the replacement of lost glands, and the regeneration of specialised cells within intact glands. In the latter situation, the stem-cell compartment is preserved and removal of an injurious factor could lead to regeneration of parietal and chief cells and full restoration of function. This has been clearly demonstrated in an animal model where withdrawal of a drug that induced selective loss of parietal cells was followed by complete restitution of the oxyntic mucosa [20]. Where glands and their associated stem cells have been completely destroyed, replacements would have to arise from adjacent intact pit-gland units. In the developing mammalian stomach, multiplication of oxyntic glands occurs through a process of budding, duplication, fission and separation [21]. Whether or not a similar process occurs in the adult is debatable. It seems clear that most regeneration following gland loss involves the MNC lineage but there is evidence, albeit from a small number of subjects, to indicate that full restoration of oxyntic glands can follow atrophy [22]. When atrophy is combined with IM, the scope for reversal is further limited. In IM, the pit-gland units are replaced by neo-crypts in which the stem cell compartment is situated, as in the normal intestine, at the base of the crypt. While budding of intestinalised crypts is a distinct possibility, it would be highly unlikely to give rise to normally arranged oxyntic glands, and would merely lead to expansion of the metaplastic foci.

IM is more likely be reversible if it develops as an adaptation to an adverse factor that can be identified and removed. For instance, cytokines from chronic inflammatory cells and in particular Th2 helper lymphocytes may be responsible for "adaptive" IM in *H. pylori* infection [23]. Certainly intestinal cells cannot be colonised by the organism and will therefore enjoy a survival advantage. However, IM can have other causes (*e.g.* bile reflux, high salt diet, and alcohol) some of which may be acting synergistically. This means that even in *H. pylori*-infected subjects, factors other than infection could be provoking or accelerating the metaplastic change. If IM is a consequence of stable somatic mutations in stem cells, changes in the immediate mucosal environment may not achieve reversal. While somatic mutation could be a factor in all types of IM it is interesting that the genetic lesions found in type III IM are similar to those found in gastric dysplasia (intra-epithelial neoplasia) [16, 18, 24]. These findings cast further doubt on the potential reversibility of this particular subtype of IM. Even when IM is a consequence of epigenetic changes, for example those resulting from methylation of genes involved in cell differentiation [25], the scope for reversal may be strictly limited.

The relationships between gastritis, atrophy and IM and their potential for reversibility are illustrated in *Figure 1*.

Does reversal of atrophy and intestinal metaplasia occur?

There are several impediments to the proper assessment of reversibility, which include failings in histological interpretation, sampling errors and "spontaneous regression". When there is deep infiltration of the glandular layer by chronic inflammatory cells, separation

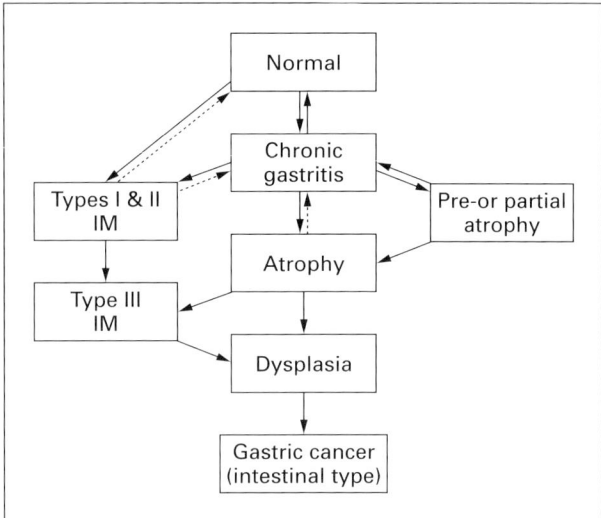

Figure 1. Hypothetical relationships between atrophy, IM and gastritis. While the reversibility of gastritis and pre- or partial atrophy to normality has been established, the reversibility of types I and II intestinal metaplasia and fully-developed glandular atrophy by eradication of *H. pylori* is unproven. Reversibility of type III metaplasia and dysplasia is considered highly unlikely.

of the glands can produce a spurious impression of atrophy. Resolution of inflammation subsequent to eradication of *H. pylori* will lead, over several months, to a return to normal gland density. This is not reversal of atrophy but histological misinterpretation. Likewise the assumption that a few small mucosal samples are representative of the whole is highly suspect when dealing with multifocal processes. Thus there are inherent difficulties in comparing atrophy and IM between baseline and follow-up endoscopies. Finally, even in the absence of treatment, all follow-up studies on chronic gastritis show apparent regression in a minority of subjects. In a large cohort follow-up study in Colombia [26], "regression" rates for the change from atrophy to normal (or superficial gastritis) and from IM to atrophy were 7.5 and 4.4/100 person-years respectively. While there was a net overall *progression*, the importance of sampling errors in giving rise to these results was emphasised.

Given that sampling errors will always confound histological interpretation, it might be thought that indirect measures of atrophy would offer a more accurate estimate, but this approach is also flawed. It is now clearly established that hypochlorhydria and changes in serum pepsinogen I and II ratios can result from corpus inflammation alone [27]. Thus some patients with profound hypochlorhdria show a substantial increase in acid output after eradication of *H. pylori* attributable to resolution of inflammation and not to regeneration of oxyntic glands [28].

Sampling errors are even more problematic in the assessment of IM. However, targeted biopsies from the margins of peptic ulcers and the subsequent "scar" clearly demonstrate that IM (usually of types I and II) frequently develops in regenerating epithelium and regresses with time [29].

Does *Helicobacter pylori* eradication suffice?

With the realisation that *H. pylori* plays a central role in gastric carcinogenesis, the notion of intervention by eradication of infection has become increasingly attractive. The elimination of inflammation will have its own beneficial consequences but can atrophy and IM be expected to regress?

The published studies looking at the reversibility of atrophy and IM in chronic *H. pylori* gastritis following eradication treatment have yielded conflicting results *(Table I)*. Regression of atrophy has been recorded in a minority of studies but only after at least a year of follow-up and then only in the antrum. Similar inconsistency characterises the possible regression of IM, and the majority of studies reveal no significant change.

Table I. Studies which have examined the possible reversal of atrophy and IM by eradication of *H. pylori* arranged according to the length of follow-up

Authors	Atrophy	Intestinal metaplasia	Length of follow-up
El-Omar *et al.*, 1997 [27]	No	No	6m
Annibale *et al.*, 2000 [30]	No	No	6m
Iijima *et al.*, 2000 [28]	No	No	7m
Genta *et al.*, 1993 [31]	–	Yes[a, c]	1y
Wittemann *et al.*, 1995 [32]	No	No	1y
van der Hulst *et al.*, 1997 [33]	No	No	1y
Schenk *et al.*, 2000 [34]	Yes[a]	No	1y
Sung *et al.*, 2000 [35]	No	Yes[a]	1y
Satoh *et al.*, 1998 [36]	No	No	1-3.25y
Forbes *et al.*, 1996 [37]	No	No	7y

Only studies which have been published as full papers in peer-reviewed journals are listed.
[a] = antrum, [c] = corpus mucosa

Substantial benefit in terms of regression of these premalignant conditions is claimed in the first reported randomised intervention trial of the effects of *H. pylori* eradication and dietary supplementation with vitamin C or β-carotene [38]. This was carried out in a high-incidence gastric cancer region (in Colombia) on 852 infected subjects who had atrophic gastritis and/or IM at entry and who were biopsied at 36 and 72 months following intervention treatment. The authors concluded that the elimination of *H. pylori* produced "a marked and statistically significant increase in the rate of regression of the precursor lesions". But similar relative risks were obtained for the other treatments alone, and, as Blot has pointed out [39], it is disturbing that anti-*H. pylori* treatment was effective when given alone but conveyed no (added) benefit when given with vitamin C or β-carotene. Although the results are promising, Blot concluded that in view of the lack of consistency, the findings should be interpreted with caution. Perhaps further caution is called for when it is appreciated that a change from IM at baseline to multifocal atrophic gastritis at follow-up qualifies as "regression" according to their histological protocol.

While true regression of atrophy and IM will depend upon the capacity of the mucosa to regenerate specialised glandular tissue, at least proper identification and elimination of the cause could be expected to prevent progression. However, it is clear that atrophy and IM have a number of causes – bile reflux, dietary irritants and autoimmunity, as well as *H. pylori* infection. Removal of infection may therefore be insufficient to produce reversal.

It seems most likely that regeneration of normal oxyntic glands following true glandular atrophy with replacement fibrosis will be, at least, limited. Likewise restoration of normal differentiation in IM is improbable in the presence of stable mutations in stem cells. In effect, certain forms of atrophy and IM have passed a "point of no return" and reversal becomes impossible. In my view, the hope that intervention by elimination of *H. pylori* will of itself lead to substantial reversal of atrophy and IM is an unrealistic expectation. However, a more realistic outcome has been established already. *H. pylori* eradication leads to resolution of inflammation, elimination of DNA damage by reactive oxygen species, a reduction in cell turnover, a rise in acid output in hypochlorhydric subjects, and a gradual return of ascorbic acid secretion into the gastric juice. These proven consequences could be much more important in the prevention of gastric cancer than the hoped-for reversal of atrophy and IM.

Acknowledgements

This article is a slightly expanded version of a leading article published by *Gut* (Prospects for intervention in gastric carcinogenesis: reversibility of gastric atrophy and intestinal metaplasia. *Gut* 2001; 49: 2-4).

References

1. Correa P, Haenszel W, Cuello C, Archer M, Tannenbaum S. A model for gastric cancer epidemiology. *Lancet* 1975; ii: 58-60.
2. Asaka M, Kato M, Kudo M, *et al*. Atrophic changes of gastric mucosa are caused by *Helicobacter pylori* infection rather than aging: studies in asymptomatic Japanese adults. *Helicobacter* 1996; 1: 52-6.
3. DeLuca VA, West AB, Haque S, *et al*. Long-term symptom patterns, endoscopic findings, and gastric histology in *Helicobacter pylori*-infected and uninfected patients. *J Clin Gastroenterol* 1998; 26: 106-12.
4. Maaroos HI, Vorobjova T, Sipponen P, *et al*. An 18-year follow-up study of chronic gastritis and *Helicobacter pylori* association of *CagA* positivity with development of atrophy and activity of gastritis. *Scand J Gastroenterol* 1999; 34: 864-9.
5. Stolte M, Baumann K, Bethke B, *et al*. Active autoimmune gastritis without total atrophy of the glands. *Z Gastroenterol* 1992; 30: 729-35.
6. Claeys D, Karapetian O, Saraga M, *et al*. Mouse mammary tumor virus superantigens and murine autoimmune gastritis. *Gastroenterology* 1994; 107: 924-33.

7. Sakagami T, Dixon M, O'Rourke J, et al. Atrophic gastric changes in both *Helicobacter felis* and *Helicobacter pylori* infected mice are host dependent and separate from antral gastritis. *Gut* 1996; 39: 639-48.
8. Schmidt PH, Lee JR, Joshi V, et al. Identification of a metaplastic cell lineage associated with human gastric adenocarcinoma. *Lab Invest* 1999; 79: 639-46.
9. Hanby AM, Poulsom R, Playford RJ, Wright NA. The mucous neck cell in the human gastric corpus: a distinctive, functional cell lineage. *J Pathol* 1999; 187: 331-7.
10. Farinati F, Cardin R, Degan P, et al. Oxidative DNA damage accumulation in gastric carcinogenesis. *Gut* 1998; 42: 351-6.
11. Claeys D, Faller G, Appelmelk BJ, Negrini R, Kirchner T. The gastric H^+, K^+-ATPase is a major autoantigen in chronic *Helicobacter pylori* gastritis with body mucosa atrophy. *Gastroenterology* 1998; 115: 340-7.
12. Slack JMW. Epithelial metaplasia and the second anatomy. *Lancet* 1986; ii: 268-71.
13. Slack JMW. Stem cells in epithelial tissues. *Science* 2000; 287: 1431-3.
14. James RJ. Homeodomain proteins and cell phenotype. *Gastroenterology* 1997; 113: 680-6.
15. Silberg DA, Furth EE, Taylor JK, Schuck T, Chiou T, Traber PG. CDX1 protein expression in normal, metaplastic, and neoplastic human alimentary tract epithelium. *Gastroenterology* 1997; 113: 478-86.
16. Tahara E. Molecular biology of gastric cancer. *World J Surg* 1995; 19: 484-8.
17. Ochiai A, Yamauchi Y, Hirohashi S. p53 mutations in the non-neoplastic mucosa of the human stomach showing intestinal metaplasia. *Int J Cancer* 1996; 69: 28-33.
18. Hamamoto T, Yokozaki H, Semba S, et al. Altered microsatellites in incomplete-type intestinal metaplasia adjacent to primary gastric cancers. *J Clin Pathol* 1997; 50: 841-6.
19. Wu MS, Shun CT, Lee WC, et al. Gastric cancer risk in relation to *Helicobacter pylori* infection and subtypes of intestinal metaplasia. *Br J Cancer* 1998; 78: 125-8.
20. Goldenring JR, Ray GS, Coffey RJ, et al. Reversible drug-induced oxyntic atrophy in rats. *Gastroenterology* 2000; 118: 1080-93.
21. Hattori T, Fujita S. Fractographic study on the growth and multiplication of the gastric gland of the hamster. *Cell Tiss Res* 1974; 153: 145-9.
22. Oberhuber G, Wuendisch T, Rappel S, Stolte M. Significant improvement of atrophy after eradication therapy in atrophic body gastritis. *Path Res Pract* 1998; 194: 609-13.
23. Ishikawa N, Wakelin D, Mahida YR. Role of T helper 2 cells in intestinal goblet cell hyperplasia in mice infected with *Trichinella spiralis*. *Gastroenterology* 1997; 113: 542-9.
24. Tahara E. Carcinogenesis and progression of human gastric cancer. *Trans Soc Pathol Jpn* 1993; 119: 265-72.
25. Sugimura T, Ushijima T. Genetic and epigenetic alterations in carcinogenesis. *Mutat Res* 2000; 462: 235-46.
26. Correa P, Haenszel W, Cuello C, et al. Gastric precancerous process in a high risk population: cohort follow-up. *Cancer Res* 1990; 50: 4737-40.
27. El-Omar EM, Oien K, El-Nujumi A, et al. Helicobacter pylori infection and chronic gastric acid hyposecretion. *Gastroenterology* 1997; 113: 15-24.
28. Iijima K, Ohara S, Sekine H, et al. Changes in gastric acid secretion assayed by endoscopic gastrin test before and after *Helicobacter pylori* eradication. *Gut* 2000; 46: 20-6.
29. Silva S, Filipe MI, Pinho A. Variants of intestinal metaplasia in the evolution of chronic atrophic gastritis and gastric ulcer. A follow up study. *Gut* 1990; 31: 1097-104.
30. Annibale B, Aprile MR, D'ambra G, et al. Cure of *Helicobacter pylori* infection in atrophic body gastritis patients does not improve mucosal atrophy but reduces hypergastrinemia and its related effects on ECL-cell hyperplasia. *Aliment Pharmacol Ther* 2000; 14: 625-34.
31. Genta RM, Lew GM, Graham DY. Changes in the gastric mucosa following eradication of *Helicobacter pylori*. *Mod Pathol* 1993; 6: 281-9.

32. Witteman EM, Mravunac M, Becx MJCM, Hopman WPM, Verschoor JSC, Tytgat GNJ, de Koning RW. Improvement of gastric inflammation and resolution of epithelial damage one year after eradication of *Helicobacter pylori*. *J Clin Pathol* 1995; 48: 250-6.
33. van der Hulst RWM, van der Ende A, Dekker FW, *et al*. Effect of *Helicobacter pylori* eradication on gastritis in relation to *cagA*: a prospective 1-year follow-up study. *Gastroenterology* 1997; 113: 25-30.
34. Scenk BE, Kuipers EJ, Nelis GF, *et al*. Effect of *Helicobacter pylori* eradication on chronic gastritis during omeprazole therapy. *Gut* 2000; 46: 615-21.
35. Sung JY, Lin SR, Ching JY, *et al*. Atrophy and intestinal metaplasia one year after cure of *H. pylori* infection: A prospective, randomized study. *Gastroenterology* 2000; 119: 7-14.
36. Satoh K, Kimura K, Takimoto T, Kihira K. A follow-up study of atrophic gastritis and intestinal metaplasia after eradication of *Helicobacter pylori*. *Helicobacter* 1998; 3: 236-40.
37. Forbes GM, Warren JR, Glaser ME, *et al*. Long-term follow-up of gastric histology after *Helicobacter pylori* eradication. *J Gastroenterol Hepatol* 1996; 11: 670-3.
38. Correa P, Fontham ETH, Bravo JC, *et al*. Chemoprevention of gastric dysplasia: Randomized trial of antioxidant supplements and anti-Helicobacter pylori therapy. *J Natl Cancer Inst* 2000; 92: 1881-8.
39. Blot WJ. Preventing cancer by disrupting progression of precancerous lesions. *J Natl Cancer Inst* 2000; 92: 1868-9.

Primary sclerosing cholangitis: prevention and/or specific therapy

Siegfried Wagner, Peter N. Meier, Michael P. Manns

Department of Gastroenterology and Hepatology, Medizinische Hochschule Hannover, Hannover, Germany

Primary sclerosing cholangitis (PSC) is a chronic cholestatic liver disease of unknown etiology, commonly associated with inflammatory bowel disease. It is characterized by inflammation, destruction and fibrosis of intrahepatic and extrahepatic bile ducts [1, 2]. The natural history of PSC is characterized by remissions and exacerbations, frequently terminating in cirrhosis and liver failure [3, 4]. No currently accepted specific therapy exists for this disease, and liver transplantation is the only life-extending therapeutic alternative for patients with end-stage PSC. The aim of this chapter is to give an overview on the current state of the management of PSC and its complications.

Pathogenesis

To take measures for prevention of PSC implies that the pathogenesis of the disease is understood. Unfortunately, the etiology of PSC has remained widely elusive. Several theories have been suggested to explain the development of PSC, such as autoimmunity, portal bacteriemia, absorption of colonic toxins, ischemic injury, viral infections, toxic bile acids, and genetic predisposition [2, 5-12]. Several cellular and humoral immune mechanisms support the concept of an immunologic disturbance as the underlying cause of PSC. There is an aberrant expression of HLA class II and ICAM-1, and an increased expression of heat shock protein 65 (hsp65) on biliary epithelium [10, 13]. PSC patients frequently have elevated serum levels of immunoglobulins and a variety of non-organ-specific autoantibodies. These abnormalities seem to reflect merely markers of immune reactions occurring in this condition, and some may be associated with underlying IBD if present. Antinuclear antibodies and anti-smooth muscle antibodies occur in less than half of patients with PSC, whereas antimitochondrial antibodies are almost never found [2]. A cytoplasmic antineutrophil antibody (pANCA) detected in a high proportion of patients with PSC may also be detected in serum from patients with other autoimmune liver diseases such as autoimmune hepatitis and PBC [14-16]. Antibodies directed against shared epitopes on biliary and colonic epithelium may provide a more direct causal link in patients with chronic ulcerative colitis and PSC [17]. Genetic susceptibility in PSC patients is based on the association with certain HLA genotypes, like HLA DRB1*0301 (DR3) and DRB3*0101 (DRw52a) alleles, whereas the DRB1*0401 (DR4) allele may be a marker of more rapid disease progression [18, 19]. The aberrant expression of class II HLA antigen on bile duct epithelium may be secondary to biliary obstruction and not an underlying event. The strong association between PSC and IBD has suggested portal bacteriemia as a potential antigen source in genetically predisposed individuals which may lead to activation of Kupffer cells in the liver with the consequent increased production of tumor necrosis factor. PSC, however, may exist without any evidence of IBD; it may present several years before the bowel disease or a long time after colectomy, and colectomy is not associated with any effect on the course of PSC [2]. Very recent findings suggest an association between mutations in one allele of the cystic fibrosis transmembrane conductance regulator (CFTR) gene and PSC. The carrier state for CFTR mutations may predispose to the development of PSC in patients with IBD.

Management of primary sclerosing cholangitis

Medical treatment

At this time, no established medical therapy is available that alters the progressive course of PSC. Promising, but variable results have been obtained with ursodeoxycholic acid (UDCA) therapy [20-26]. In most trials, UDCA at doses varying from 10 to 15 mg/kg/d has been shown to improve liver biochemistries, whereas liver histology has been reported to improve infrequently. In the largest randomized, controlled trial of UDCA (13-15 mg/kg/d), there was improvement in laboratory tests in patients randomized to UDCA relative to those in the placebo group, but this was not accompanied by beneficial changes in clinical outcomes after up to 6 years of follow-up [24]. Higher doses of UDCA (25-30 mg/kg/d) in the treatment of PSC look promising and are now under evaluation in large, controlled trials [26]. Other drugs that have not been found effective include penicillamine, methotrexate, colchicine, cyclosporine, tacrolimus, nicotine, and pentoxifylline [2, 27-30]. At this time, although there is no proven therapy for slowing or reversing the primary disease process, medical therapy of PSC patients with UDCA (10-15 mg/kg/d) has been recommended by experts of a national consensus panel [31]. Patients with decompensated liver cirrhosis or hyperbilirubinemia (> 15 mg/dl) should be excluded.

Medical measures in the treatment of complications of PSC are aimed at providing relief from pruritus, correcting nutritional deficiencies (especially fat-soluble vitamin deficiency), and the treatment and prevention of bacterial cholangitis. The cause of pruritus is unknown. Symptomatic treatment is started with oral cholestyramine, 4 to 8 g three times daily just before meals. In addition, general skin care with topical emollients (lanolin, menthol ointments) is recommended. Antihistamines are effective in some patients. Refractory pruritus may be treated with opiate antagonists like naloxone and nalmefene or 5-HT3 antagonists like ondansetrone. Fat-soluble vitamins (A, D, E, K) should be substituted regularly. Osteopenic bone disease has been reported in PSC patients, but is less frequent than in PBC patients [32-34]. Besides substitution of deficiencies in vitamin D and calcium, antiresorptive agents such as biphosphonates (etidronate, pamidronate, alendronate) may be beneficial. Episodes of bacterial cholangitis may be caused by infestation with Gram-negative bacilli, enterococci, bacteroides, and clostridia, and should be treated with ciprofloxacin alone, or a combination of mezlocillin or a third generation cephalosporin with metronidazole. Long-term antibiotic prophylaxis has been shown not to alter the natural history of PSC. In some patients with recurrent episodes of cholangitis, intermittent antibiotic prophylaxis may be indicated, but an indication for liver transplantation should also be considered.

Endoscopic treatment

ERCP plays a central role in the management of PSC. Cholangiography is not only the gold standard for diagnosis of PSC but it gives also some information on the prognosis of the disease. High grade strictures and diffuse strictures of the intrahepatic ducts have been identified as indicators of poor prognosis [35]. ERCP is also of importance in the evaluation and management of complications of PSC. In the follow-up of PSC patients, diagnostic cholangiography is indicated if recurrent cholangitis develops or if there is a rapid deterioration of liver function. Therapeutic endoscopic measures are required if there are bile duct stones or dominant strictures of the major bile ducts. ERCP is a safe method for establishing the diagnosis of PSC in asymptomatic patients (2% complication rate); although ERCP in symptomatic patients carries a higher risk (14%), this can be justified by the benefits of endoscopic therapy [36].

Endoscopic treatment modalities in PSC patients include hydrostatic balloon dilatation of strictures, removal of ductal exsudates and debris, nasobiliary perfusion, and intermittent placement of endoprosthesis. An endoscopic treatment of biliary stenoses in PSC is indicated if focal dominant strictures of the extrahepatic bile duct including the right and left hepatic duct are suspected, and if there is evidence of cholestasis [37-40]. This condition implies that only a minority of PSC patients will be suited for endoscopic therapy representing about 20-30% of PSC patients [41]. Diffuse intrahepatic strictures cannot be treated endoscopically.

For the reopening of dominant bile duct stenoses, endoscopic dilation therapy is especially suited. Angioplasty-type balloon catheters allow application of high pressure (10-12 bar) at a defined outer diameter (5-10 mm). Coaxial dilators are helpful in very tight strictures where a balloon catheter cannot be passed. For long-lasting reopening of biliary strictures by dilation therapy multiple treatment sessions are necessary [35-39]. Endoscopic placement of endoprosthesis is an alternative method for management of biliary strictures. Stenting provides an immediate biliary drainage, especially in high grade strictures. The main problem of endoprostheses is the recurrent occlusion of the stents associated with bacterial cholangitis [42]. Therefore stents should be removed or changed within 4 weeks [31, 43]. Another endoscopic treatment modality in PSC is biliary lavage by nasobiliary perfusion. This allows removal of biliary exsudate and debris, and is usually combined with dilation therapy.

Table I summarizes the treatment strategy of the Medizinische Hochschule Hannover for management of biliary strictures in PSC patients. All patients receive antibiotic prophylaxis. If dominant strictures are identified and endoscopic therapy is planned, we routinely perform a sphincterotomy to facilitate insertion of the ballon catheter and to separate the bile duct orifice from the pancreas thereby minimizing the risk of complicating pancreatitis. A guide wire is placed into the stenotic bile duct and an angioplasty catheter is advanced through the stricture under fluoroscopic control. Dilatation is performed by serial inflations of the balloon with physiological saline (supplemented with contrast medium) up to a maximum pressure of 10 bar *(Figure 1)*. If multiple dominant strictures are present, each of them may be treated during one session. Subsequently, a nasobiliary catheter is inserted through the most proximal dominant stricture into an intrahepatic portion of the biliary system for irrigation (500-1000 ml/day). After irrigating the biliary tree for one week, balloon dilatation is repeated. Our preference is not to place an endoprosthesis because of frequent stent occlusion and the development of complicated bacterial cholangitis. However, in case of unsuccessful reopening of strictures by balloon dilation stent placement is indicated. All patients continue treatment with UDCA.

Table I. Endoscopic therapy of biliary strictures in primary sclerosing cholangitis: procedure and follow-up

---

- Antibiotic prophylaxis (ciprofloxacin or mezlocillin)
- Endoscopic sphincterotomy of the papilla
- Dilation with angioplasty-type balloon catheter under fluoroscopic guidance
  - 6-10 mm outer diameter
  - inflation with contrast medium diluted with saline, at a pressure of 12 bar
  - procedure repeated until complete reopening of the stricture
- Nasobiliary catheter perfusion (normal saline 500-1000 ml/d) for 1 week
- Repeat balloon dilation after 1 week
- Cholangiographic follow-up at 3 to 12 months intervals, repeat dilation if necessary
- Stent placement only if dilation treatment is unsuccessful
- Continuation of UDCA treatment

Table II summarizes the outcome and the major characteristics of PSC patients treated with different endoscopic measures. The interpretation of the results of these studies is hampered by the varying study designs and the different endoscopic treatment modalities applied. Up to now, no randomized controlled trials have been published on endoscopic treatment of PSC patients. Nonetheless, the published data clearly show that endoscopic therapy is beneficial in selected patients. In these trials follow-up varied between 23 and 52 months; overall about 60-80% showed an improvement of clinical, cholangiographic, and laboratory data. In two studies an improved survival of treated PSC patients was observed when compared with the predicted survival using the Mayo Clinic survival model [40, 44]. It may be concluded from current data that endoscopic treatment is effective and safe in selected patients with dominant strictures of the major bile ducts.

The main problem in the follow-up of PSC patients is the recognition of developing cholangiocarcinoma which may occur in 10-15% of PSC patients [3, 4, 45-47]. The autopsy prevalence of cholangiocarcinoma is even higher. Patients with complicating biliary malignancy have an extremely poor prognosis, even if the carcinoma is incidentally found during liver transplantation. Up to now there is no reliable way to distinguish a dominant

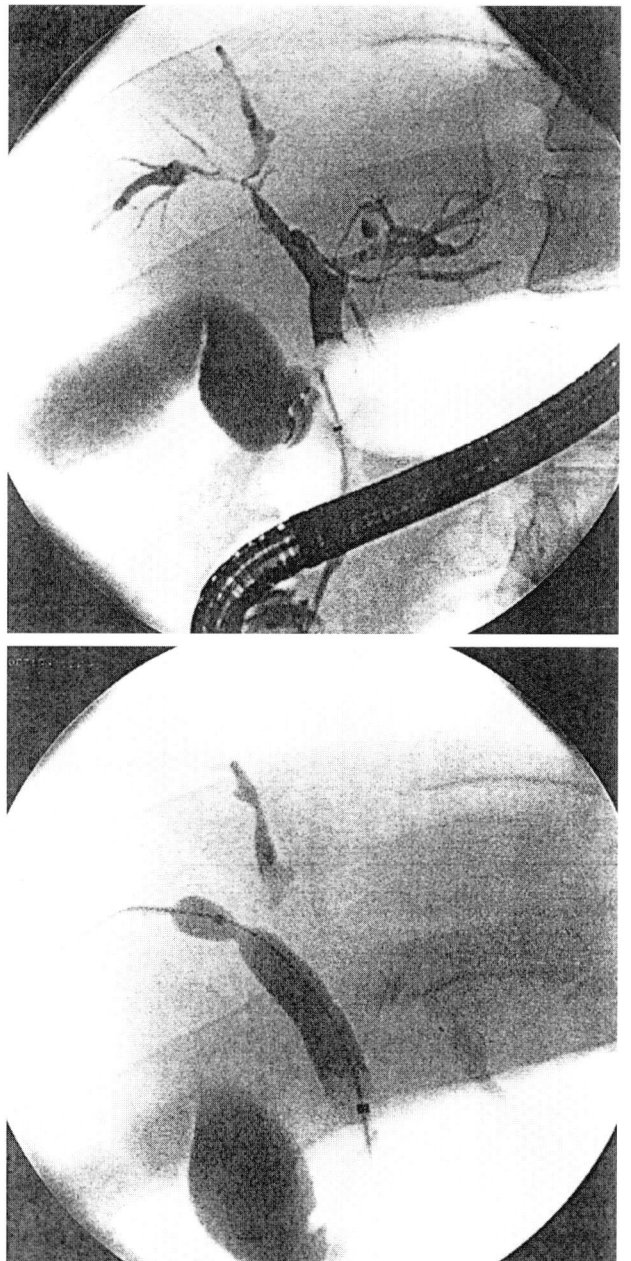

Figure 1. Cholangiograms of a PSC patient with focal strictures of the main intrahepatic ducts (adapted from Meier PN, Manns MP. *Best Practice and Research Clinical Gastroenterology* 2001, in press).
a. Occlusion cholangiogram. b. Balloon dilatation of a dominant stricture of the right hepatic duct.

Table II. Outcome of primay sclerosing cholangitis patients on endoscopic therapy: review of the literature

• Baluyut *et al.* [40]	
• prospective study	n = 63
• procedure	ballon dilation
• follow-up	34 months
• outcome	improved survival compared to predicted rates
• Ponsioen *et al.* [43]	
• prospective study	n = 32
• procedure	short-term stent therapy
• follow-up	4 years
• outcome	reintervention-free 80% and 60% at 1 and 3 years, respectively
• Stiehl *et al.* [44]	
• prospective study	n = 23
• procedure	balloon dilation and UDCA therapy
• follow-up	45 months
• outcome	improved survival compared to predicted rates
• Wagner *et al.* [39]	
• prospective study	n = 12
• procedure	balloon dilation and UDCA therapy
• follow-up	23 months
• overall improvement	75%
• van Milligen de Wit *et al.* [54]	
• retrospective study	n = 25
• procedure	stent therapy
• follow-up	29 months
• asymptomatic after Rx	57%
• Lee *et al.* [38]	
• retrospective study	n = 53
• procedure	dilation, stenting, nasobiliary tube
• follow-up	31 months
• overall improvement:	77%
• Gaing *et al.* [37]	
• retrospective study	n = 42
• procedure	dilation, stenting, nasobiliary perfusion
• follow-up	52 months
• biochemical improvement:	70%
• Johnson *et al.* [55]	
• retrospective study	n = 35
• procedure	dilation (stenting)
• follow-up	24 months
• overall improvement:	85%

stricture from a cholangiocarcinoma. Brush cytology may identify malignancy, and new methods such as intraductal ultrasound (IDUS), cholangioscopy, and PET may have a role in the future.

Surgical treatment

The role of biliary surgery in PSC has diminished considerably with the growing success of liver transplantation [2]. Prior biliary surgery may complicate liver transplantation [48-52]. Therefore, biliary surgery in patients with PSC should be minimized and reserved for selected noncirrhotic patients who have marked cholestasis or recurrent cholangitis caused by a dominant extrahepatic or hilar stricture not amenable to endoscopic dilatation. Currently, liver transplantation is the only life-extending therapeutic alternative for patients with end-stage PSC. Long-term outcome in liver transplanted PSC patients is good, with 5-year survival rates ranging between 57% and 89% [50, 51, 53]. The question of recurrent PSC in the allograft is difficult to answer, but its incidence is probably low (< 10%).

Conclusion

PSC is an increasingly recognized chronic cholestatic liver disease of unknown cause which is characterized by a slow but relentless progress leading to cirrhosis and liver failure. No specific treatment for PSC currently exists, although ursodiol has some beneficial effects. Liver transplantation is the treatment of choice for patients with advanced liver disease. Endoscopic treatment is indicated in symptomatic patients with dominant strictures of the major bile ducts. Repeated angioplasty-type balloon dilatation and short-term endoscopic placement of endoprosthesis are the treatment of choice for biliary stenoses. Endoscopic therapy results in a sustained reopening of biliary strictures which leads to an improvement of clinical, cholangiographic, and biochemical findings in the majority of selected patients. Early detection of complicating cholangiocarcinoma remains a diagnostic challenge.

References

1. Lee YM, Kaplan MM. Primary sclerosing cholangitis. *N Engl J Med* 1995; 332: 924-33.
2. Angulo P, Lindor KD. Primary sclerosing cholangitis. *Hepatology* 1999; 30: 325-32.
3. Farrant JM, Hayllar KM, Wilkinson ML, Karani J, Portmann BC, Westaby D, et al. Natural history and prognostic variables in primary sclerosing cholangitis. *Gastroenterology* 1991; 100: 1710-7.
4. Broome U, Olsson R, Loof L, Bodemar G, Hultcrantz R, Danielsson A, et al. Natural history and prognostic factors in 305 Swedish patients with primary sclerosing cholangitis. *Gut* 1996; 38: 610-65.
5. Minuk GY, Angus M, Brickman CM, Lawley TJ, Frank MM, Hoofnagle JH, et al. Abnormal clearance of immune complexes from the circulation of patients with primary sclerosing cholangitis. *Gastroenterology* 1985; 88: 166-70.
6. Lindor KD, Wiesner RH, LaRusso NF, Homburger HA. Enhanced autoreactivity of T-lymphocytes in primary sclerosing cholangitis. *Hepatology* 1987; 7: 884-8.
7. Jorge AD, Esley C, Ahumada J. Family incidence of primary sclerosing cholangitis associated with immunologic diseases. *Endoscopy* 1987; 19: 114-7.
8. Mieli-Vergani G, Lobo-Yeo A, McFarlane BM, McFarlane IG, Mowat AP, Vergani D. Different immune mechanisms leading to autoimmunity in primary sclerosing cholangitis and autoimmune chronic active hepatitis of childhood. *Hepatology* 1989; 9: 198-203.

9. Fausa O, Schrumpf E, Elgjo K. Relationship of inflammatory bowel disease and primary sclerosing cholangitis. *Semin Liver Dis* 1991; 11: 31-9.
10. Boberg KM, Lundin KE, Schrumpf E. Etiology and pathogenesis in primary sclerosing cholangitis. *Scand J Gastroenterol* Suppl. 1994; 204: 47-58.
11. Wiesner RH. Current concepts in primary sclerosing cholangitis. *Mayo Clin Proc* 1994; 69: 969-82.
12. van Milligen de Wit AW, van Deventer SJ, Tytgat GN. Immunogenetic aspects of primary sclerosing cholangitis: implications for therapeutic strategies. *Am J Gastroenterol* 1995; 90: 893-900.
13. Adams DH, Hubscher SG, Shaw J, Johnson GD, Babbs C, Rothlein R, *et al.* Increased expression of intercellular adhesion molecule 1 on bile ducts in primary biliary cirrhosis and primary sclerosing cholangitis. *Hepatology* 1991; 14: 426-31.
14. Duerr RH, Targan SR, Landers CJ, LaRusso NF, Lindsay KL, Wiesner RH, *et al.* Neutrophil cytoplasmic antibodies: a link between primary sclerosing cholangitis and ulcerative colitis. *Gastroenterology* 1991; 100: 1385-91.
15. Seibold F, Weber P, Klein R, Berg PA, Wiedmann KH. Clinical significance of antibodies against neutrophils in patients with inflammatory bowel disease and primary sclerosing cholangitis. *Gut* 1992; 33: 657-62.
16. Klein R, Eisenburg J, Weber P, Seibold F, Berg PA. Significance and specificity of antibodies to neutrophils detected by western blotting for the serological diagnosis of primary sclerosing cholangitis. *Hepatology* 1991; 14: 1147-52.
17. Das KM, Vecchi M, Sakamaki S. A shared and unique epitope(s) on human colon, skin, and biliary epithelium detected by a monoclonal antibody. *Gastroenterology* 1990; 98: 464-9.
18. Olerup O, Olsson R, Hultcrantz R, Broome U. HLA-DR and HLA-DQ are not markers for rapid disease progression in primary sclerosing cholangitis [see comments]. *Gastroenterology* 1995; 108: 870-8.
19. Mehal WZ, Lo YM, Wordsworth BP, Neuberger JM, Hubscher SC, Fleming KA, *et al.* HLA DR4 is a marker for rapid disease progression in primary sclerosing cholangitis. *Gastroenterology* 1994; 106: 160-7.
20. O'Brien CB, Senior JR, Arora Mirchandani R, Batta AK, Salen G. Ursodeoxycholic acid for the treatment of primary sclerosing cholangitis: a 30-month pilot study [published erratum appears in *Hepatology* 1992 Mar; 15: 566]. *Hepatology* 1991; 14: 838-47.
21. Beuers U, Spengler U, Kruis W, Aydemir U, Wiebecke B, Heldwein W, *et al.* Ursodeoxycholic acid for treatment of primary sclerosing cholangitis: a placebo-controlled trial. *Hepatology* 1992; 16: 707-14.
22. Lebovics E, Salama M, Elhosseiny A, Rosenthal WS. Resolution of radiographic abnormalities with ursodeoxycholic acid therapy of primary sclerosing cholangitis. *Gastroenterology* 1992; 102: 2143-7.
23. Gross JB, Jr. Promises, promises: ursodeoxycholic acid for primary sclerosing cholangitis. *Gastroenterology* 1993; 104: 941-3.
24. Lindor KD. Ursodiol for primary sclerosing cholangitis. Mayo Primary Sclerosing Cholangitis-Ursodeoxycholic Acid Study Group. *N Engl J Med* 1997; 336: 691-5.
25. van Hoogstraten HJ, Wolfhagen FH, van de Meeberg PC, Kuiper H, Nix GA, Becx MC, *et al.* Ursodeoxycholic acid therapy for primary sclerosing cholangitis: results of a 2-year randomized controlled trial to evaluate single *versus* multiple daily doses. *J Hepatol* 1998; 29: 417-23.
26. Harnois DM, Angulo P, Jorgensen RA, LaRusso NF, Lindor KD. High-dose ursodeoxycholic acid as a therapy for patients with primary sclerosing cholangitis. *Am J Gastroenterol* 2001; 96: 1558-12.
27. Knox TA, Kaplan MM. A double-blind controlled trial of oral-pulse methotrexate therapy in the treatment of primary sclerosing cholangitis [see comments]. *Gastroenterology* 1994; 106: 494-9.
28. Olsson R, Broome U, Danielsson A, Hagerstrand I, Jarnerot G, Loof L, *et al.* Colchicine treatment of primary sclerosing cholangitis. *Gastroenterology* 1995; 108: 1199-203.

29. Van Thiel DH, Carroll P, Abu Elmagd K, Rodriguez Rilo H, Irish W, McMichael J, et al. Tacrolimus (FK 506), a treatment for primary sclerosing cholangitis: results of an open-label preliminary trial. *Am J Gastroenterol* 1995; 90: 455-9.
30. LaRusso NF, Wiesner RH, Ludwig J, MacCarty RL, Beaver SJ, Zinsmeister AR. Prospective trial of penicillamine in primary sclerosing cholangitis. *Gastroenterology* 1988; 95: 1036-42.
31. Beuers U, Wiedmann KH, Kleber G, Fleig WE. [Therapy of autoimmune hepatitis, primary biliary cirrhosis and primary sclerosing cholangitis. Consensus of the German Society of Digestive System and Metabolic Diseases]. *Z Gastroenterol* 1997; 35: 1041-9.
32. Hay JE, Lindor KD, Wiesner RH, Dickson ER, Krom RA, LaRusso NF. The metabolic bone disease of primary sclerosing cholangitis. *Hepatology* 1991; 14: 257-61.
33. Lindor KD, Janes CH, Crippin JS, Jorgensen RA, Dickson ER. Bone disease in primary biliary cirrhosis: does ursodeoxycholic acid make a difference? *Hepatology* 1995; 21: 389-92.
34. Angulo P, Therneau TM, Jorgensen A, DeSotel CK, Egan KS, Dickson ER, et al. Bone disease in patients with primary sclerosing cholangitis: prevalence, severity and prediction of progression. *J Hepatol* 1998; 29: 729-35.
35. Craig DA, MacCarty RL, Wiesner RH, Grambsch PM, LaRusso NF. Primary sclerosing cholangitis: value of cholangiography in determining the prognosis. *AJR Am J Roentgenol* 1991; 15: 959-64.
36. van den Hazel SJ, Wolfhagen EH, van Buuren HR, van de Meeberg PC, Van Leeuwen DJ. Prospective risk assessment of endoscopic retrograde cholangiography in patients with primary sclerosing cholangitis. Dutch PSC Study Group. *Endoscopy* 2000; 32: 779-82.
37. Gaing AA, Geders JM, Cohen SA, Siegel JH. Endoscopic management of primary sclerosing cholangitis: review, and report of an open series. *Am J Gastroenterol* 1993; 88: 2000-8.
38. Lee JG, Schutz SM, England RE, Leung JW, Cotton PB. Endoscopic therapy of sclerosing cholangitis. *Hepatology* 1995; 21: 661-7.
39. Wagner S, Gebel M, Meier P, Trautwein C, Bleck J, Nashan B, et al. Endoscopic management of biliary tract strictures in primary sclerosing cholangitis. *Endoscopy* 1996; 28: 546-51.
40. Baluyut AR, Sherman S, Lehman GA, Hoen H, Chalasani N. Impact of endoscopic therapy on the survival of patients with primary sclerosing cholangitis. *Gastrointest Endosc* 2001; 53: 308-12.
41. Wagner S, Meier P, Manns M. Endoscopic therapy of primary sclerosing cholangitis patients. In: Manns MP, Stiehl A, Chapman RW, Wiesner R, eds. *Primary sclerosing cholangitis*. Dordrecht: Kluwer Academic Publishers, 1997.
42. Motte S, Deviere J, Dumonceau JM, Serruys E, Thys JP, Cremer M. Risk factors for septicemia following endoscopic biliary stenting. *Gastroenterology* 1991; 101: 1374-81.
43. Ponsioen CY, Lam K, van Milligen de Wit AW, Huibregtse K, Tytgat GN. Four years experience with short term stenting in primary sclerosing cholangitis. *Am J Gastroenterol* 1999; 94: 2403-7.
44. Stiehl A, Rudolph G, Sauer P, Benz C, Stremmel W, Walker S, et al. Efficacy of ursodeoxycholic acid treatment and endoscopic dilation of major duct stenoses in primary sclerosing cholangitis. An 8-year prospective study. *J Hepatol* 1997; 26: 560-6.
45. Nashan B, Schlitt HJ, Tusch G, Oldhafer KJ, Ringe B, Wagner S, et al. Biliary malignancies in primary sclerosing cholangitis: timing for liver transplantation. *Hepatology* 1996; 23: 1105-11.
46. Rosen CB, Nagorney DM, Wiesner RH, Coffey RJ, Jr., LaRusso NF. Cholangiocarcinoma complicating primary sclerosing cholangitis. *Ann Surg* 1991; 213: 21-5.
47. Bergquist A, Glaumann H, Persson B, Broome U. Risk factors and clinical presentation of hepatobiliary carcinoma in patients with primary sclerosing cholangitis: a case-control study. *Hepatology* 1998; 27: 311-6.
48. Ahrendt SA, Pitt HA, Kalloo AN, Venbrux AC, Klein AS, Herlong HF, et al. Primary sclerosing cholangitis: resect, dilate, or transplant? *Ann Surg* 1998; 227: 412-23.
49. Farges O, Malassagne B, Sebagh M, Bismuth H. Primary sclerosing cholangitis: liver transplantation or biliary surgery. *Surgery* 1995; 117: 146-55.

50. Narumi S, Roberts JP, Emond JC, Lake J, Ascher NL. Liver transplantation for sclerosing cholangitis. *Hepatology* 1995; 22: 451-7.
51. Abu Elmagd KM, Malinchoc M, Dickson ER, Fung JJ, Murtaugh PA, Langworthy AL, *et al.* Efficacy of hepatic transplantation in patients with primary sclerosing cholangitis. *Surg Gynecol Obstet* 1993; 177: 335-44.
52. Ismail T, Angrisani L, Powell JE, Hubscher S, Buckels J, Neuberger J, *et al.* Primary sclerosing cholangitis: surgical options, prognostic variables and outcome. *Br J Surg* 1991; 78: 564-7.
53. Goss JA, Shackleton CR, Farmer DG, Arnaout WS, Seu P, Markowitz JS, *et al.* Orthotopic liver transplantation for primary sclerosing cholangitis. A 12-year single center experience. *Ann Surg* 1997; 225: 472-81.
54. van Milligen de Wit AW, van Bracht J, Rauws EA, Jones EA, Tytgat GN, Huibregtse K. Endoscopic stent therapy for dominant extrahepatic bile duct strictures in primary sclerosing cholangitis. *Gastrointest Endosc* 1996; 44: 293-9.
55. Johnson GK, Geenen JE, Venu RP, Schmalz MJ, Hogan WJ. Endoscopic treatment of biliary tract strictures in sclerosing cholangitis: a larger series and recommendations for treatment. *Gastrointest Endosc* 1991; 37: 38-43.

Dysplasia in ulcerative colitis: management principles

Jerome D. Waye

Endoscopy Unit, Mount Sinai Hospital and GI Endoscopy Unit, Lenox Hill Hospital, New York, USA

Dysplasia is an unequivocal neoplastic change in tissues [1]. It is always present in an adenoma, and is considered to be the precursor lesion of malignant development in inflammatory bowel disease (IBD). Dysplasia often, but does not always, precede the onset of malignancy in IBD. Not all dysplastic lesions progress, but it is currently believed that dysplasia may progress to carcinoma and that the changes occur over time, and usually pass through stages, from low to high grade and then to malignancy.

In ulcerative colitis and in Crohn's disease, malignancy is a feared complication. In ulcerative colitis, the tendency for malignancy is dependent upon two factors: the longevity of the inflammatory process and its extent in the colon. In ulcerative colitis, the risk begins at 8 years after onset of the inflammatory involvement and is dependent on the length of bowel involved, with the lowest risk occurring in patients with proctitis, and the highest risk in patient's with universal colonic involvement [2]. In Crohn's disease, the duration of disease activity as a precursor of malignancy is the same as in ulcerative colitis, but the risk appears to be correlated with the involvement of at least one-third the length of the large bowel [3].

Because of the progression through various degrees of dysplastic change, surveillance colonoscopy in IBD has become accepted as a tool to determine whether the colon harbors early neoplastic histology which will trigger intervention in a timely fashion to prevent the subsequent development of cancer.

For small discrete lesions, endoscopic removal of a dysplastic area may be possible, or removal of the entire colon will interrupt the dysplasia-carcinoma sequence.

There are several problems with reliance upon dysplasia for the prevention of cancer in IBD [4]. It is well known that colonoscopic surveillance may "miss" the development of carcinoma in some patients while in a surveillance program. The alternative is to remove the dysplastic areas upon making the diagnosis of dysplasia [2]. Unfortunately, about 25% of patients undergoing repeated surveillance colonoscopy will develop cancer [2]. When dysplasia is found, it tends to be multi-focal.

Therefore, endoscopic removal of small dysplastic lesions or segmental resection of dysplastic areas may not protect colon from metachronous development of dysplasia. Indeed, when dysplasia has been found in one segment of the colon, there is an 18-50% chance of having carcinoma elsewhere in the colon when surgical colectomy has been performed [2]. Another problem is that although the criteria for the pathologist to make the diagnosis of dysplasia was set out by the IBD Morphology Study Group [1], the interpretive agreement when the same slides are circulated to various pathologists is less than perfect [5]. For low-grade dysplasia, the agreement may be rather disparate. It is possible that some of the changes of low-grade dysplasia may be closely mimicked by an active inflammatory process [2]. In spite of this, the disparity in making the diagnosis of low-grade dysplasia is not paralleled in the diagnosis of high-grade dysplasia [5].

For most gastroenterologists, the pathologic criteria set up by the "Morphology Study Group" have been well accepted. When the diagnosis of "indefinite dysplasia" is received, it is usually accepted as a possibility of dysplasia, perhaps requiring closer observation. A larger problem is that although the diagnosis of "high grade dysplasia" is almost universally accepted as a trigger for intervention, gastroenterologists often take the diagnosis of "low grade dysplasia" as yet another warning signal that the patient needs to be more closely observed. The problem which engenders the most debate in the field of cancer and IBD is what approach should be taken in the patient with an unequivocal diagnosis of low-grade dysplasia. Hanauer [6] states that "if experienced pathologists confirm an interpretation of low-grade dysplasia, I recommend colectomy".

DALM's and polyps in colitis

The report by Blackstone et al. [7] that 54% of colitis patients with dysplasia in a mass lesion had cancer at surgery introduced the term "DALM" into the vocabulary of gastroenterology. The term "DALM" refers to a dysplasia-associated lesion or mass. The original description of a DALM [7] included many lesions that were already malignant, but the biopsy failed to make the diagnosis of cancer. In Blackstone's original description of twelve cases having a DALM, five were single polypoid masses varying in size from 2×2 cm up to 5×20 cm. Two were plaque-like (one of unknown size, the others 2×3 cm). In five cases, "the lesion appeared as multiple, sessile polyps confined to a 5-15 cm segment of colon". In fact, the two smaller single dysplastic polyps of 0.5 cm and 0.6-1.5 cm did not harbor any cancer. In this paper, the authors made the point that not all patients with a DALM require colectomy, specifically mentioning the "typical tubular adenoma, 1 cm or less" in a patient who falls into the expected age range (over 45 years). They state that "these lesions can be completely removed with electrosurgery, and the patients followed with repeat colonoscopy, at appropriate intervals, provided that biopsies of the surrounding flat mucosal failed to demonstrate dysplasia".

In patients with IBD with sessile polypoid lesions that have the morphologic appearance of adenomas without evidence of malignancy (ulceration, concave surface, friable or bleeding), the lesions may be removed with the wire snare and cautery technique [8]. A lesion of similar size and configuration that is probably an inflammatory polyp (smooth and shiny or with a white exudate) can be left alone. Most inflammatory polyps and adenomas have well-defined and sharp borders, but those with indistinct edges blending into adjacent mucosa are more likely to be adenomas. If the histopathologist reports the resected polyp as "dysplastic", the information should not trigger an automatic reaction to recommend surgical extirpation of the colon, since all adenomas are dysplastic, whether in the colitic or normal colon. Small lesions that the endoscopist feels are completely removed should be treated in a manner similar to adenomas in the non-colitic patient [8, 9]. However, if the lesion is irregular, extends into surrounding mucosa ("carpeting") or is part of a larger lesion that cannot be totally removed endoscopically, then the consideration should be that this is a dysplasia-associated mass, and, if it cannot be completely extirpated endoscopically, surgery should be considered. The key to whether these lesions should be treated endoscopically or not is the level of confidence of the endoscopist in determining whether the lesion is amenable to endoscopic resection and, following resection, if the endoscopist feels that the entire lesion was removed. The location of such a colitis-associated dysplastic polyp, whether in a diseased area or proximal to it, makes no difference in the final outcome of the patient [10-12].

When a discrete adenoma (dysplastic polyp) is removed from a colitic colon in an area of active or healed colitis, the colon wall adjacent to the margins of the lesion should be biopsied in an attempt to determine whether the dysplasia is a "field defect", with surrounding dysplasia in the flat adjacent mucosa [7, 8, 10]. If a field defect is found, then surgery should be considered. However, if there is no surrounding dysplasia, the lesion is discrete and totally removed endoscopically, the patient should be endoscopically followed more closely than after removal of a single adenoma in a non-colitic patient, but the pathology report of a "dysplastic lesion" in a colitic patient does not mandate a surgical colonic resection, even though the polypoid component was removed. The recent literature suggests that endoscopists must closely inspect any polypoid lesion in colitis, with particular attention to the surface, borders, adjacent mucosa and whether the polyps are solitary or multiple [8]. Engelsgjerd et al. [11] included all lesions with a discrete, well-defined sessile or pedunculated polypoid gross appearance in which clinical distinction of a coincidental sporadic adenoma was impossible. By definition, all these dysplastic lesions were histologically indistinguishable from typical sporadic adenoma. In their attempt to characterize the safety of removal of discrete adenomas, they excluded dysplastic lesions that were considered the surface of a mass or were irregular, elevated or broad-based. Both of these papers report that although other adenomas may develop in the colitic segments, there were no concerns that occurred during the follow-up interval. Odze et al. [12] considered that lesions were sporadic adenomas in patients with chronic ulcerative colitis if they were located outside (proximal) colitic involvement, since these are not thought to be chronic ulcerative colitis-related dysplastic polyps. Chronic ulcerative colitis-associated polypoid dysplastic lesions were classified as those that were located within histologically proven areas of colitis and were associated with either synchronous or metachronous flat dysplasia or adenocarcinoma.

The gastroenterologist must be aware that all adenomas are dysplastic. The dysplastic changes in the colon of IBD patients are no different from the dysplastic changes seen in an adenoma. Because of the similarity of the histopathologic features, pathologists are unable to state whether a biopsy received in the laboratory came from a flat area of bowel, a slightly elevated velvety plaque, or from a polyp. It is now accepted that in IBD, discrete dysplastic polyps that can be totally removed with the snare and cautery technique should be treated as an adenoma whether sessile or pedunculated, providing that the surrounding mucosa has been biopsied as has been shown to be non-dysplastic.

To the endoscopist, dysplasia may range from frankly polypoid masses covering large areas of mucosa to discrete slightly elevated sessile plaques, from millimeter size to several centimeters in diameter. Dysplastic areas may also appear as "warty" mucosal excrescences, often barely distinguishable from surrounding mucosa; hence the need for multiple biopsies. A 1988 review [13] indicated that dysplasia in flat mucosa as a sole marker for occult carcinoma may be less common and less predictive of carcinoma than previously thought. The St. Mark's group described the macroscopic lesions of dysplasia as nodular, irregular, elevated areas or as a sessile polyp [14] Although Cook and Goligher reported several carcinomas not recognized prior to microscopic examination [15], the St. Mark's 1983 study [16] indicated that of 52 carcinomas, 51 were associated with a visible lesion and only one occurred in flat mucosa. The 1980 study by Nugent and Haggitt [17] identified dysplasia in one of three patterns: flat mucosa, a villous surface configuration, and polypoid excrescences. A 1989 review [18] corroborated the overall impression that colonic dysplasia may be both diffuse and focal and that endoscopic recognition of dysplasia becomes feasible when the surface shows a villous or velvety nodularity. According to Riddell [19] and Dobbins [20], plaques and slightly verrucose or nodular lesions must be deliberately sought by endoscopists, since colitis-associated carcinomas may be little more than a minimally elevated plaque with either a smooth or slightly verrucous surface, sometimes no more than 1 cm in diameter.

The enigma of low-grade dysplasia

In spite of the knowledge that dysplasia, either low-grade or high-grade, is a neoplastic entity, most gastroenterologists treat the finding of low-grade dysplasia on biopsy as a warning of future events. This attitude has developed for several reasons, among which is the relatively low incidence of colon cancer associated with the finding of low-grade dysplasia on surveillance biopsies as opposed to the higher incidence of carcinoma associated with the biopsy diagnosis of high-grade dysplasia. Several authorities have suggested a "more careful" surveillance follow-up scheme for patients with low-grade dyplasia [2, 21], which many have found not to be reproducible on subsequent biopsies. However, the ability to re-biopsy six months later an area where dysplasia had previously been found, may easily miss the area of previous biopsy and create a false sense of security that low-grade dysplasia has indeed "disappeared". Some of patients whose low-grade dysplasia was not found on subsequent biopsies will develop cancer of the colon in that area, attesting to the large sampling area that occurs with surveillance biopsies in the colitis bowel. About 15% of patients in surveillance series have low-grade dysplasia, and if surgery is performed for the diagnosis of low-grade dysplasia, cancer has been found in 18% [22]. It has been estimated that 33 biopsies taken throughout the large bowel during surveillance endoscopies will give a 90% chance of finding dysplasia if it is present [23], with an increase to 95% assurance that dysplasia will be found on biopsy if it is present by taking 56 biopsies.

A significant disparity in the recommendations and in the actual practice of surveillance biopsies has been reported [24]. When gastroenterologists were requested to divulge their schema for biopsies during surveillance colonoscopy in colitis patients, it was found that about half of them take between 6 and 10 biopsies throughout the colon, with a third taking between 11 and 15. When a biopsy diagnosis of low-grade dysplasia was found, about three-quarters of the gastroenterologists will repeat the colonoscopy with 3-6 months, and if low-grade dysplasia were not present on repeat examination, routine surveillance would be recommended. Many would advise a colectomy if low-grade dysplasia were confirmed at a second colonoscopy.

When dysplasia of any grade is discovered during surveillance examination in IBD, the greatest assurance that cancer of the colon will not develop is in the total removal of the large bowel. This decision is one not readily suggested by many gastroenterologists, nor easily accepted by patients. The decision for colectomy often is a result of an agreement reached between the physician and the patient based on the findings of dysplasia. If a dysplasia associated lesion or mass is detected, and is deemed endoscopically unresectable, irrespective of the grade of dysplasia, there is probably a greater than 50% risk of that lesion being an invasive carcinoma. On the other hand, in many institutions, a single or an occasional low-grade dysplasia biopsy may not result in surgery [25].

For those who adopt a "wait and watch" response on the finding of low-grade dysplasia on surveillance biopsy, the following are the most frequent findings that suggest surgical intervention: 1) repeated low-grade dysplasia; 2) multi-focal low-grade dysplasia; 3) transformation to high-grade dysplasia.

For patients with Crohn's disease, the incidence of carcinoma is similar to that of ulcerative colitis for patients with long-standing disease (over 8 years) and with more than one-third of the colon involved with an inflammatory process [3]. Here, surveillance biopsies are considered to be as indicated as in patients with chronic ulcerative colitis.

Practical advice

The term "dysplasia" in ulcerative colitis often generates a knee-jerk reflex that surgery should be performed. However, the histological diagnosis of dysplasia is often not a hard and firm conclusive reading. This is especially true of the diagnosis of low-grade dysplasia. Because of the fluidity of the diagnosis, most gastroenterologists opt for repeating the biopsies in an attempt to confirm the histology and prevent unnecessary surgery. The difficulty with this approach is sampling error and the reported findings of cancer in some colons removed for a finding of low-grade dysplasia. As for discrete dysplastic lesions, their removal is sufficient therapy (regardless of patient age) providing that the lesion is totally resected and that biopsies of surrounding and distant areas are negative for dysplasia. It is true that any adenoma is a lesion or a mass, and that these are dysplastic, but the acronym has been interpreted over the years to mean that the finding of a DALM mandates surgery. The true significance of the dysplastic lesion will depend upon its morphology, completeness of removal, and biopsies of surrounding tissue. Neither the pathologist nor the endoscopist should have their reports interpreted as isolated bits of information. To reach the correct conclusion, the input of both specialists is required.

References

1. Riddell RH, Goldman H, Ransohoff DF, et al. Dysplasia in inflammatory bowel disease; standardized classification with provisional clinical applications. *Hum Pathol* 1983; 14: 931.
2. Ahman DJ. In: Kirsner JB, ed. *Gastrointestinal malignancies in inflammatory bowel*, 5th ed. Philadelphia : W.B. Saunders, 2000: 379-94.
3. Friedman S, Rubin PH, Bodian C, Goldstein E, Harpaz N, Present DH. Screening and surveillance colonosocpy in chronic Crohn's colitis. *Gastroenterology* 2002; 120: 820-6.
4. Ransohoff D, Riddell RH, Levin B. Ulcerative colitis and colonic cancer: problems in assessing the diagnosis usefulness of mucosal dysplasia. *Dis Colon Rectum* 1985; 28: 383.
5. Eaden J, Abrams K, McKay H, Denley H, Mayberry J. Inter-observer variation between general and specialist gastrointestinal pathologists when grading dysplasia in ulcerative colitis. *Pathol* 2002; 194: 152-7.
6. Hanauer SB. Surveying surveillance, Editorial. *Gastrointest Endosc* 2000; 51: 240-2.
7. Blackstone M, Riddell R, Rogers BHG, Levin B. Dysplasia-associated lesion or mass (DALM) detected by colonoscopy in long-standing ulcerative colitis: an indication for colectomy. *Gastroenterology* 1981; 80: 366-74.
8. Rubin PH, Friedman S, Harpaz N, Goldstein E, Weiser J, Schiller J, Waye JD, Present DH. Colonoscopic polypectomy in chronic colitis: conservative management after endoscopic resection of dysplastic polyps. *Gastroenterology* 1999; 177: 1295-300.
9. Medlicott SA, Jewell LD, Price L, Fedorak RN, Sherbaniuk RW, Urbanski SJ. Conservative management of small adenomata in ulcerative colitis. *Am J Gastroenterol* 1997; 92: 2094-8.
10. Torres C, Antonioli D, Odze RD. Polypoid dysplasia and adenomas in inflammatory bowel disease. *Am J Surg Pathol* 1998; 22: 275-84.
11. Engelsgjerd M, Farraye FA, Odze RD. Polypectomy may be adequate treatment for adenoma-like dysplastic lesions in chronic ulcerative colitis. *Gastroenterology* 1999; 117: 1288-94.
12. Odze RD. Adenomas and adenoma-like DALMs in chronic ulcerative colitis: a clinical, pathological and molecular review. *Am J Gastroenterol* 1999; 94: 1746-50.
13. Isbell G, Levin B. Ulcerative colitis and colon cancer. *Gastroenterol Clin North Am* 1988; 17: 773.
14. Lennard-Jones J, Ritchie J, Morson B, et al. Cancer surveillance in ulcerative colitis. *Lancet* 1983; 2: 149.
15. Cook M, Goligher J. Carcinoma and epithelial dysplasia complicating ulcerative colitis. *Gastroenterology* 1975; 68: 1127-30.
16. Butt J, et al. Macroscopic lesions in dysplasia and carcinoma complicating ulcerative colitis. *Dig Dis Sci* 1983; 28: 18-20.
17. Nugent F, Haggit R. Long-term follow-up, including cancer surveillance, for patients with ulcerative colitis. *Clin Gastroenterol* 1980; 9: 459-61.
18. Albert M, Nochomovitz L. Dyplasia and cancer surveillance in inflammatory bowel disesase. *Gastroenterol Clin North Am* 1989; 18: 83.
19. Riddell R. Endoscopic recognition of early carcinoma in ulcerative colitis. *JAMA* 1977; 237: 2811.
20. Dobbins W. Dysplasia and malignancy in inflammatory bowel disease. *Rev Med* 1984; 35: 33.

21. Canto MI, Petras RE, Sivak MV, Jr. Problems in IBD. In: Sivak MV, ed. *Gastroenterologic Endoscopy*, 2nd ed. Philadelphia: W.B. Saunders, 2000: 1306-23.
22. Woolrich AJ, DaSilva MD, Korelitz BI. Surveillance in the routine management of ulcerative colitis: the predictive value of low-grade dysplasia. *Gastroenterology* 1992; 103: 431.
23. Rubin CE, Haggift RC, Brentnall TA, *et al*. DNA aneuploidy in colonic biopsies predicts future development of dysplasia in ulcerative colitis. *Gastroenterology* 1992; 103: 611.
24. Eaden JA, Ward BA, Mayberry JF. How Gastroenterologists Screen for Colonic Cancer in Ulcerative Colitis: An Analysis of Performance. *Gastrointest Endosc* 2000: 51: 123-8.
25. Lewin KJ, Riddell RH, Weinstein WM. *Dysplasia in IBD*. New York: Igaku-Shoin, 1992: 933-51.

II

Novel Techniques for Gastrointestinal Tumour Removal

Mucosectomy: new therapeutic strategy in case of high grade intraepithelial neoplasia and early cancer of the upper GI-tract

C. Ell

Department of Internal Medicine II, Wiesbaden, Germany

Summary

In the Western countries, endoscopic experience of local endoscopic therapy of early cancers in the upper GI-tract is still relatively low, since the incidence of early stomach cancer is lower than in Japan and generally operable patients with early cancer will be referred to surgery for radical resection. This situation changes now slowly since the number of detected early malignant lesions, especially in the lower esophagus, increases rapidly and the techniques of mucosectomy in junction with other endosopic methods as photodynamic therapy and thermal techniques offer a broad spectrum of methods for curative endoscopic treatment in carefully selected patients with malignant or premalignant lesions in the esophagus and stomach.

The incidence of adenocarcinoma of the esophagus has increased continuously during the last decades. Chronic acid reflux is strongly associated with adenocarcinoma of the esophagus and is the main cause of the development of specialised intestinal metaplasia in the esophagus (Barrett's esophagus). Barrett's esophagus is therefore considered a precancerous condition. Published data on malignant transformation in Barrett's esophagus show rates varying between 1 in 46 and 1 in 141 patients/years. More recent prospective data show that in Barrett's esophagus with histologically proven severe dysplasia adenocarcinoma subsequently develops in up to 34%.

The treatment of choice with curative intent has been esophagectomy. However, even at surgical centres that have sufficient experience and even, when patients are selected carefully, the mortality rates are in the range of 3% and 5% with Barrett's early carcinoma (EC) and high-grade intraepithelial neoplasia (HGN), respectively. There is a significant morbidity rate ranging from 18% to 48%. In view of these facts and because of the relatively large proportion of patients who are unable to undergo surgery because of comorbidity or age, the question arises whether local endoscopic therapy might also be applicable in Barrett's EC and HGN, in analogy with early gastric cancer. Arguments in favour of intraluminal treatment by means of endoscopic techniques are as follows: morbidity and mortality should be essentially lower than in esophagectomy. With endoscopic techniques, there is no major loss of quality of life. Furthermore, there are no risks for lymph node metastases in proven HGN and the risk for lymph nodes metastases is almost zero in patients with mucosal Barrett's cancer. Preliminary data negate that in analogy to early gastric cancer, the lymph node metastases risk is very low, too (probably 1-2%) in patients with Barrett's carcinoma from the submucosa level-I-type (SM 1 cancer). However, the lymph node metastases rate ranges between 10% and 20% in submucosal cancer of the 2nd and 3rd level (SM 2 and SM 3 cancer).

Staging procedures

In consequence, in all patients with malignant or pre-malignant lesions in the stomach and esophagus carefully designed staging procedures are necessary to find out preoperatively the patients with low risk for lymph node metastases, if local endoscopic treatment is scheduled. The staging procedures include – at least in our specialised centre – high-resolution video endoscopy with mapping biopsies, chromoendoscopy with methylen blue and biopsies of unstained or discoloured lesions. A standard endosonografy with 7.5 to 12 mHz is performed to detect lymph node enlargements in the mediastinum and the truncus coeliacus. In addition to mini-endosonografy with through-the-scope probes with 20 mHz to investigate the infiltration depth of the tumour.

Abdominal ultrasound and spiral computed tomography of the thorax/mediastinum and the upper abdomen are oncological standards.

In some cases, additional endoscopic mucosal resection is used for diagnostic purposes to get a clear information about the infiltration depth. Drug-induced or auto-fluorescence endoscopy are still experimental diagnostic methods.

The aims of the staging procedures are the exact mapping of the whole organ; that means, detection of synchronous lesions, measurement of the diameter of the malignant lesion and furthermore description of the tumour surface as a polypoid (type I), flat (type II a, b, c) or ulcerated (type III). Concerning the infiltration depth, we want to differentiate between mucosal type, submucosal type I, submucosal type II and III and, finally T2 tumours. Another important aim of the staging procedure is to get information about the tumour grading (G1 – G3). This classification of early stomach cancer is well established for already many years by the Japanese society of endoscopy.

In analogy to early gastric cancer, we hope to define "low-risk Barrett's carcinoma" and HGN as follows: uni-locular lesions smaller than 2 cm, surface type I or II, infiltration type M or SM I, grading type G1 or G2 and lymph status negative.

Endoscopic treatment techniques

Three principle endoscopic treatment techniques are available: endoscopic mucosal resection (EMR), photodynamic therapy (PDT) and thermoablation techniques as lasers and electrocoagulation. Details of the different treatment options can be obtained by the cited literature at the end of the manuscript.

Without any doubt, the treatment technique of choice has become nowadays – also in Europe – EMR: the advantages of EMR in comparison with all other local endoscopic techniques are obvious. The histological preparation of the resected specimen provides information on the depth of the invasion of the individual wall layers and allows a resection within healthy margins (Ro). If there is at the lateral margin a R1 situation, further EMRs are possible. Only when there is a R1 resection at the basal margin and/or there is a infiltration of the submucosal layer surgical resection is mandatory.

There are a couple of different EMR techniques published and possible [1-3]. In type I lesions (polypoid lesions), especially in the stomach, EMR can be performed as a standard polypectomy. Generally prior EMR injection of diluted epinephrine/saline solution can be generally recommended, especially when resecting in the stomach.

The breakthrough in EMR – especially in the esophagus – was the development of the so-called "suck and cut" technique. The easiest way was first described by the Sohendra group [3]. However, this technique did not find large acceptance yet, since the specimen resected are clearly smaller than with the other "such and cut" techniques: the cap technique with a special EMR snare developed by Inoue *et al.* [2] allows large volume resection in a one step procedure; that means there is no removing and reintroducing of the endoscope necessary.

Another possibility is to use a variceal ligation set: in a first step, the lesions is sucked in the ligation cylinder and will be ligated. Then the scope is removed and without the ligation device re-introduced. In the second step, a conventional snare is used to resect the artificially produced polyp. For the ligation technique, single use ligation sets or the re-usable so-called Euroligator are available. The latter one makes EMR remarkably cheaper, especially when a center has a high EMR frequency. Currently we have gained experience with both techniques in a prospective randomized study comparing the single use Inoue cap technique and the re-usable ligation EMR technique in 120 patients. Parts of the results are presented during the oral presentation.

Since all the treatment modalities have advantages and disadvantages (see literature), one should use a differentiated choice of the local treatment. Actually, we are using the EMR in about 60%, the PDT in about 20% and both, PDT in combination with EMR, in about 20%. Thermal methods should only be used for optimising the local endoscopic treatment and not as initial treatment.

Results

The complication rate of EMR appears in experienced hands surprisingly low. In our own experience in more than 500 EMRs in the esophagus and stomach morbidity is not higher than 2%, mortality is less than 0,2%. Smaller bleedings after resection are with 10% common, however in almost all cases the bleeding stopped spontaneously or after endoscopic injection therapy or in rare cases after clip application. Only in exceptional cases blood transfusions were required. In our experience the bleeding risk appears to be higher after EMR in the stomach than in the esophagus. In all we have seen only two perforations; one had to be operated, the other could be treated successfully by conservative therapy. Concerning EMR treatment of early cancer of the stomach there are numerous publications of Japanese and other Asian gastroenterologists. The most recent papers are cited [4, 5]. However up to now there is no larger report published in a peer-reviewed journal from a European or US center.

Actually there are only few published data on local endoscopic therapies of Barrett's EC and HGN. Publications from Asia are missing since the Barrett problem does not exist really in Asia. Besides of same small casuistic series, there are only two groups with larger experiences: the Overholt group in USA reported on 100 patients with mainly high-grade neoplasia (> 70% HGN), treated exclusively by photodynamic therapy with hematoporphyrine derivates as photosensitizer. They achieved a local remission rate of about 80%, however, the rate of major complications was 34% and consisted of strictures of the esophagus which had to be treated by repeated dilation. In 1998, our own group reported about 32 patients with HGD and EC using amino levulinic acid. Due to the high concentration of the photosensitizer only in the mucosa and the short retention time in the body, severe side effects were never observed. However, the tumour destruction by this kind of PDT is limited to a maximum of 2 mm tissue depth. This circumstance was reflected by the results: we achieved a 100% complete remission rate in HGD but only 75% complete remission rate in EC. In the meantime we gathered experience with 70 patients altogether, treated by PDT (results not yet published).

Last year, our group published a larger experience in endoscopic mucosal resection (*Gastroenterology* 2000; 118: 670-7): prospective investigation of EMR was conducted in 64 patients (61 patients with EC and 3 patients with HGD); 35 patients met the criteria for low risk. A total of 120 EMR was performed with only 1 major complication. A spurting bleeding could be managed endoscopically. Complete local remission was achieved significantly earlier in the low-risk group than in the high-risk group. A complete remission was achieved in 97% (34/35) of the patients in the low-risk group. In the high-risk group the complete remission rate was lower (59%). However, life table analyses showed that in this group a similar complete remission rate can also be expected after completion of all therapeutic steps.

Updated results of 114 out of 157 patients, who were treated locally in our center within the last 3 years (10/1996 – 9/1999), showed a complete remission rate of 98%. Only 2 patients suffered treatment failures and were treated by esophagectomy. The rate of major complications was 0% in this series. During the follow-up of 18 months (mean) in 26 patients metachronous lesions were detected and treated by endoluminal techniques again (the actual results are not yet published).

Conclusions

Without any doubt, radical surgical resection is still the treatment of choice for superficial malignant lesions in the upper GI-tract, especially when they are located in the esophagus. In Europe, local endoscopic methods or intraluminal therapy are still experimental. However, the concept of local treatment is attractive because of the low morbidity, low mortality and the preservation of quality of life.

The data from Asia are generally excellent even concerning the long term follow up. They support the idea of local endoscopic curative treatment in early malignancies of the upper GI-tract. However, the question is still open whether it is allowed to transfer 1:1 the data from Asia to Europe.

However, also the first data currently available from European centers for intraluminal surgery show an excellent acute and intermediate complete remission rate. In any case, more reports from different centers with a larger number of patients and long-term results have to be expected until gastrectomy and especially esophagectomy will become the method of reserve.

References

1. Ell C, May A, Gossner L, Pech O, Günter E, Mayer G, Henrich R, Vieth M, Müller H, Seitz G, Stolte M. Endoscopic mucosal resection of early cancer and high-grade dysplasia in Barrett's esophagus. *Gastroenterology* 2000; 118: 670-7.
2. Takeshita K, Inoue H, Sakei I. Endoscopic treatment of early esophageal and gastric cancer. *Gut* 1997; 40: 123-7.
3. Sohendra N, Binmoeller KF, Bohnacker S. Endoscopic snare mucosectomy in the esophagus without any additional equipment. *Endoscopy* 1997; 29: 380-2.
4. Ida K, Nakazawa S, Hiki Y, Kurihara M. A prospective study on endoscopic resection of early stomach cancer in Japan. *Digestive Endosc* 2000; 12: 19-24.
5. Miyata M, Yokoyama Y, Joh T, Seno K, Itoh M. What are the appropriate indications for endoscopic mucosal resection in early stomach cancer? *Endoscopy* 2000; 32: 773-8.
- Gossner L, Stolte M, Sroka R, Rick K, May A, Hahn EG, Ell C. Photodynamic ablation of high-grade dysplasia and early cancer in Barrett's esophagus by means of 5-aminolevulinic acid. *Gastroenterology* 1998; 114: 448-55.
- Gossner L, May A, Stolte M, Seitz G, Hahn EG, Ell C. KTP laser destruction of dysplasia and early cancer in columnar-lined Barrett's esophagus. *Gastrointest Endosc* 1999; 49: 8-12.

Transgastric endoscopic approaches

H. Lönnroth

Sahlgrenska University Hospital, Göteborg, Sweden

With the introduction of videoimaging for endoscopy and laparoscopy the range of minimally invasive procedures that substitute open surgical techniques has rapidly increased. Removal of gastric polypes or small superficial gastric malignancies by snare cauterisation constitutes some of the most effective endotherapeutic manœuvres performed currently. The development of laparoscopy and advanced laparoscopic instruments has further provided means to gain access to not only the abdominal cavity but also to the lumen of hollow viscera. During the last 20 years a large number of different ways to gain access to the gastric lumen through direct and indirect techniques have been presented. These techniques have made it possible for several authors to present case reports as well as consecutive series of patients treated with different minimal invasive techniques for different types of gastric tumour.

Techniques for endoluminal surgery

Obviously access to the inside of the stomach can be reached with the gastroscope and through this route an endoscopically guided percutaneous endoscopic gastrotomy (PEG) as initially described by Ponsky *et al.* [1] can easily be accomplished. Through the PEG channel a direct access to the stomach with laparoscopic instruments further increases the possibility to perform intragastric interventions with minimally invasive surgical techniques. Gastroscopically guided direct introduction of trocars for laparoscopy into the gastric lumen had been described as well as indirect access to the stomach through laparoscopic route.

Tools for direct endoluminal surgery

Without the use of standard laparoscopy it is possible to gain access to the stomach without introduction of gas into the abdominal cavity. To prevent risk of leak from the opening of the stomach wall it is possible to do percutaneous anchoring of the anterior stomach wall to the anterior peritoneum by means of percutaneously introduced T-fasteners (Wilson-Cook Medical GI Endoscopy). The use of 2 mm micro-endoscopes and microinstruments as well as the of radialy expanding diameter trocars (RED trocars, Innerdyne) is the risk of bleeding as well ass leaks. Through a 5 mm PEG port ultrasound scissors can be used for intraluminal dissection. These techniques have been used by a number of intra, and transgastric procedures such as pancreatic cystogastrostomy; it was first presented by Way in 1994 [2]. Since his first report Way has presented nine cases with the use of RED trocars and T-fasteners that enabled him to open pancreatic pseudocysts through the posterior stomach wall and continuing into the cystic cavity for debris extraction and resection of multiple cyst walls. This has also been presented by Gagner [3] and others.

Laparoscopic assisted intraluminal gastric excision

Endoscopic polypectomy is an accepted standard method for moving polypes from the stomach. Complications include polypectomy bleeding (1-7%) and persistent ulceration (4-18) [4]. With the use of electocautery using electrosnare it is also possible to excise early gastric cancer as described by a number of Japanese authors [5]. Tada *et al.* injected 5 mm of saline solution into the submucosa of the gastric lesion to elevate it. The lesion was then grasped with forceps and resected using a electrosnare. This technique of so-called endoscopic mucosa resection (EMR) has, however, some limitations. Using electrocautery damages the tissue for several mm at the line of resection. Therefore, complete excision may be uncertain. Moreover excision of excessive tissue may lead to acute or delayed perforation of the stomach wall.

Further development of laparoscopic intraluminal gastric surgery has been presented by Ohashi *et al.* [6] for the first time in 1994. Ohashi reported a series of eight patients: six with early gastric cancer, one with submucosal leiomyoma and one with a giant polyp of the stomach [7]. The technique for introduction of trocars into the stomach was similar to that as described by Way [2]. In addition to this also a nasogastric tube with a balloon was placed in the duodenum and the balloon was inflated to prevent CO_2 gas flow from the stomach to the small intestine. Adequate mucosal resection was performed by dissecting the mucosal margin with electrocautery, forceps, or laser. No intraoperative or postoperative complications were reported. Another report from Ohgami *et al.* [8] presents a five year experience with 61 consecutive cases who were diagnosed with mucosal gastric cancer and were successfully treated with two different laparoscopic techniques; intragastric mucosal resection or laparoscopic wedge resection. Of the 61 patients 17 were treated with laparoscopic intragastric mucosal resection for lesions of the posterior wall of the stomach and near the cardia or the pylorus. Indications for these treatments have been: 1) preoperatively diagnosed mucosal cancer, 2) < 25 mm diameter elevated lesions and 3) < 15 mm diameter depressed lesions without ulcer formation. There were no conversions to open surgery in the series and no interoperative complication or mortality. Ulcer formation was observed in the area of resection of the stomach after surgery in all patients, but it was usually epithelialised in 4-6 weeks. At the histological examination the procedures were regarded curative. One recurrence has been reported after 2 years. This was a localised small lesion that was successfully treated by endoscopic laser irradiation.

Laparoscopic wedge resection

In the report of Ohgami [8] the majority of patients (44 out of 61 patients) were treated with a lesion lifting technique with a laparoscopic wedge resection. For the lesion lifting method marking clips were placed around the cancerous lesion during preoperative gastroscopy. The sites of the marking clips were confirmed by the cancer negative biopsies. The area on the stomach when this method was used was the anterior wall, the lesser curvature, and the greater curvature of the stomach. The wedge resection was performed with traditional laparoscopy with introduction of pneumoperitoneum. The location of the cancerous lesion was confirmed with the assistance of intraoperative gastroscopy. The gastric wall in the vicinity of the lesion was pierced by 12-gauge sheathed needle. Through this a metal rod similar to the T-fastened technique enabled the phycisian to elevate the lesion and precisely resect it with a multifire endoscopic stapling device. Of the 44 patients treated with laparoscopic wedge resection the cancerous infiltration was limited to the mucosal layer without lymphatic or venous invasion in 42 cases. Slight cancerous invasion of the submucosal layer was found in 2 cases. One of these patients also had lymphatic invasion and underwent total gastrectomy with lymph node dissection (D3) four weeks after initial surgery. One recurrency is reported. It occurred near the staple line two years after initial surgery and this patient underwent open gastrectomy.

PEG assisted endoscopic mucosal resection

A combined technique of gastroscopy and the use of a PEG-port has been described by Murai *et al.* [9]. Six patients with early gastric cancer were treated with endoscopic mucosal resection (EMR). Forceps are introduced through a PEG-port and used to grasp the lesion and thus facilitate the use of electrosnare introduced through the gastroscope. All patients were treated successfully.

Transgastric Buess endoscopic technique

This technique with the use of the 40 mm Buess endoscope through a open gastrotomy has been described by Yamashita *et al.* [10]. This technique includes a mini laparotomy where the stomach wall is lifted up to the abdominal wall incision, sutured to the skin and the 40-mm Buess scope introduced through the gastrotomy. Results have been presented from six patients with early gastric cancer, two cases of atypical epithelium, and one case of ectopic pancreas. Full thickness resection through the endoscope was also performed in four cases of leiomyomas. All lesions were resected endoluminally and the postoperative course in all cases was uneventful. Obviously the technique is suited for posterior wall lesions of the stomach. A number of different case reports including gastrointestinal stromacell tumours have been reported. Nine patients with posterior gastric stroma tumour were treated through a laparoscopic gastrotomy by Hepworth et al. [11]. In this consecutive series 9 patients with posterior gastric stromal tumours were treated with laparoscopic gastrotomy. The tumour was delivered through the gastrotomy into the abdominal cavity and excised with a linear cutter. Two patients required conversion since their tumour could not be delivered into the abdominal cavity.

Discussion

Development of surgical instruments and endoscopic videoimaging has made it possible to develop a number of different minimally invasive surgical techniques for resection of full thickness or partial thickness organ walls. Surgical contra-indications are similar to those by standard laparoscopy namely former surgery with extensive adhesions, massive ascites, coagulopathy etc. Other contra-indications and limitations are more related to the controversy of the short-term benefits *vs* the absolute goal of curative surgery and minimum of recurrence of tumour. Selection criteria for early gastric cancer have been stated by Ohgami (above). Another controversy may be the laparoscopic treatment of gastrointestinal stroma cell tumours. Preoperative histological characterisation of nodal and well defined tumours such as leiomyomas may be difficult. Gastrointestinal stromal tumours are known for wide variability in clinical behaviour and for difficulty in determining malignancy and prognosis. Today, surgery remains the primary treatment modality for patients with GIST, but the extent of resection, including regional lymph nodes or adjacent organs, remains unclear. Along with variability of the management of these patients, this difficulty in classifying GIST contribute to a wide variation in reported five years survival rates. In a retrospective review of 70 patients with gastrointestinal stromal cell tumours Pierie *et al.* [12] concluded that a complete gross surgical resection is presently the only means of cure for GIST. This has to be taken into account in the laparoscopic treatment of tumours preoperatively judged as leiomyomas.

Furthermore, histological irradiation is effective by use of electrocautery in minimal invasive surgery. Several mm of the margins of the patients may be destroyed by the electric energy. The use of ultrasound scissors, cutting staples and wide margins of stomach wall resection may limit the risk of non curative resections. Staining with methylene blue injection further improves the localisation of the tumours. In the future combined techniques with endoscopic or laparoscopic ultrasound and combination of high resolution endoscopy and laparoscopy may further improve the accuracy of the minimally invasive techniques.

References

1. Ponsky JL, Gauderer MW. Percutaneous endoscopic gastrostomy: a nonoperative technique for feeding gastrostomy. *Gastrointest Endosc* 1981; 27: 9-11.
2. Way LW, Legha P, Mori T. Laparoscopic pancreatic cystgastrostomy: the first operation in the new field of intraluminal laparoscopic surgery. *Abstract Surg Endosc* 1994; 8: 235.
3. Gagner M. Laparoscopic treatment of cystic tumors and cysts of the pancreas. In: Brune I, ed. *Laparo-endoscopic surgery*. Berlin: Blackwell Publishing, 1995: 143-6.
4. Yasuda K, Nakajima M, Kawai K. Endoscopic diagnosis and treatment of early gastric cancer. *Gastrointest Endosc Clin North Am* 1992; 2: 495-8.
5. Tada M, Shimada M, Yanai H, Tada M, Shimada M, Yamai H, Arima K, Karita M, Okazaki K, Takemoto T, Kimoshita Y, Kimoshita K, Iida Y, Watanabe H. A new technique of gastric biopsy. *Stomach Intest* 1984; 19: 1107-10.
6. Ohashi S, Yoden Y, Kanno H, Akashi A. "Laparoscopic intragastric surgery" with interventional endoscopy: a new concept in laparoscopic surgery. (Abstract) *Surg Endosc* 1994; 8: 497-9.
7. Ohashi S. Laparoscopic intraluminal (intragastric) surgery for early gastric cancer: a new concept in laparoscopic surgery. *Surg Endosc* 1995; 9: 169-71.
8. Ohgami M, Otani Y, Kumai K, Kubota T, Kim YI, Kitajima M. Curative laparoscopic surgery for early gastric cancer: Five years experience. *World J Surg* 1999; 23: 187-93.
9. Murai R, Ando H, Mitsumori N, Hada T, Fuijioka S, Nagayama A, Itsubo K. Our technique of percutaneous transgastric wall endoscopic mucosal resection, PTEMR, for early gastric cancer. (Abstract) *Surg Endosc* 1995; 10: 213.
10. Yamashita Y, Maekawa T, Sakai T, Shirakusa T. Transgastrostomal endoscopic surgery for early gastric carcinoma and for submucosal tumor. (Abstract). *Surg Endosc* 1996; 10: 267.
11. Hepworth CC, Menzies D, Motson RW. Minimally invasive surgery for posterior gastric stromal tumors. *Surg Endosc* 2000; 14: 349-53.
12. Pierie JP, Choudry U, Muzikansky A, Yeap BY, Souba WW, Ott MJ. The effect of surgery and grade on outcome of gastrointestinal stromal tumors. *Arch Surg* 2001; 136: 383-9.

Transanal endoscopic microsurgery in the treatment of rectal tumors

E. Lezoche[1], M. Guerrieri[2]

[1] II Clinica Chirurgica, Policlinico Umberto I, "La Sapienza" University, Roma, Italy
[2] Clinica di Chirurgia Generale, Ospedale Umberto I, University of Ancona, Ancona, Italy

Transanal endoscopic microsurgery (TEM) was introduced into the clinical practice by G. Buess in 1983 [1]. This technique allows the local excision of rectal adenomas and early stages of rectal cancer, well and moderately well differentiated, that have a low rate of regional spread and therefore may be treated by conservative therapy [2-5]. The TEM method utilizes a modified rectoscope allowing a three-dimensional vision of the operative field and combines all benefits of the other minimally invasive techniques: low operative trauma, less pain, reduced morbidity, faster recovery time and absence of skin scars [6].

The indications for TEM local excision are the rectal lesions located until 25 cm from the anal verge [6]

In our experience of 301 patients operated by TEM, we used two different protocols for benign and malignant tumors. Each patient underwent routine laboratory tests, an accurate clinical examination and pancolonoscopy with multiple macrobiopsies of the lesion to define histology and tumor grading.

We performed multiple biopsies of flat lesions with irregular margins and of recurrent tumors. The normal surrounding tissue was spotted with indian ink and identified by a reference number to mark the free margin around the rectal tumor [5].

Endoluminal ultrasound (EUS) was performed in tumors located within 12 cm from the anus [7] (B e K Company, Naerum, Denmark). Preoperative rigid rectoscopy was essential to measure the distance of the tumor from the anal verge and circumferential tumor spread. Moreover, it allowed us to define the feasibility of a TEM operation in tumors located beyond the rectal valves of Houston. The position of the patient (lithotomy, prone or lateral decubitus) for TEM was selected in relationship to the location of the tumor *(Figures 1, 2, 3)*.

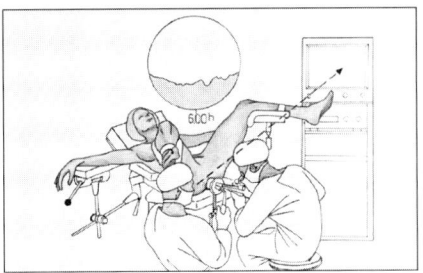

Figure 1. Position of the patient on the operative table for lesions located on the posterior wall of the rectum.

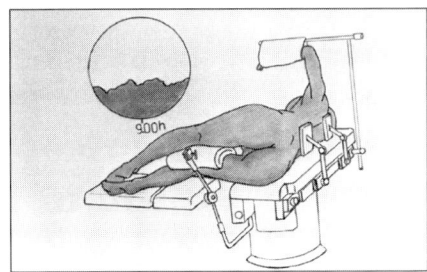

Figure 2. Lateral decubitus of the patient for lesions located on the lateral wall of the rectum.

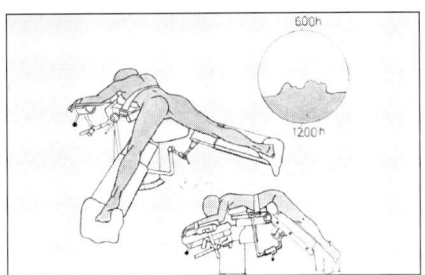

Figure 3. Prone position of the patient for lesions located on the anterior wall.

If clinical, endoscopic examination and histology were suggestive of a **benign tumor** restricted to the mucosa, as seen by endoluminal ultrasound (for lower tumors), a TEM procedure was performed without submitting the patient to other diagnostic procedures.

On the other hand, if a **malignant lesion** was suspected, the diagnostic protocol consisted of a magnetic resonance imaging (MR), which we felt was a requisite to stage rectal carcinomas preoperatively and/or of computerized tomography (CT) [8]. In malignant lesion, we considered mandatory to perform macrobiopsies for a correct assessment of the tumor grading. Moreover before radiotherapy, we performed 6-8 biopsies, marked with an india ink tattoo, one cm around the tumor margin.

Given the local nature of the excision, it is essential to obtain informed consent and to warn the patient about the oncological aspects of this method and possible complications, such as bleeding, suture dehiscence, temporary gas and/or stool incontinence, and also that a laparotomy with colonic resection or colostomy may have to be carried out if deemed necessary.

According to the preoperative diagnoses and staging, six groups of lesions can be considered elegible for TEM treatment

1. Sessile adenomas of the rectum and lower sigmoid colon within 25 cm from the anus.

2. Well and moderately well differentiated pT1 carcinomas of the extraperitoneal rectum.

3. Well and moderately well differentiated pT2 carcinomas, in patients over 75 years of age, in the extraperitoneal rectum, associated with preoperative radiotherapy.

4. pT2 or pT3 tumors, in patients at high risk for major surgery (ASA 3-4), of the extraperitoneal rectum, associated with preoperative radiotherapy.

5. pT2 or pT3 tumors in patients that refused an abdomino-perineal resection (APR), associated with preoperative radiotherapy.

6. Chronic rectal ulcerations, carcinoid tumors and endometriosis.

In rectal cancer, until April 1994, we started a preTEM radiotherapy approach consisted of 5,040 cGy, divided over 5 weeks, following after 40 days by the local excision.

An orthograde lavage of the colon and short term antibiotic prophylaxis (cephalosporin and metronidazole) were performed in all patients, preoperatively.

TEM was usually performed under general anesthesia; regional anesthesia was employed in selected cases in relationship to the physical status classification of the patient (ASA).

A 12 or 20 cm long rectoscope (external diameter 4 cm) was used (Wolf Company, Tuttlingen, Germany). The rectoscope was fixed to the operative field by a Martin arm, a supporting instrument with two joints wich maintains the required position of the instrument inside the rectum. A working insert was connected with sealing elements to prevent gas loss when the correct position of the rectoscope was obtained in relation to the location of the lesion. The optical system consisted of a three dimensional stereoscope with a bidimensional 40° angle lens connected to a video system.

An electrosurgical knife, a neddle holder, forceps, clip applicator and suction device (providing both suction and coagulation) were employed in the procedure. Recently, was used a new multifunctional instrument equipped with the functions of suction, rinsing, monopolar high frequency coagulation and bipolar high frequency dissection (ICC 350, ERBE Company, Tubingen, Germany) [9, 10].

Water was automatically injected through the rectoscope so as to clean the lens and the operative field throughout the procedure. An endosurgical unit controlled carbon dioxide insufflation, dilating the rectum with a constant measurement of endoluminal pressure.

The position and the angle of the rectoscope inside the rectum was essential to the feasibility of TEM. Usually the rectoscope was positionned with an angle of 45° in relationship to the location of the polyp *(Figure 4)*. In case of tumors located near or beyond the valves of Houston, we inserted a flexible rectoscope into the rectum beyond the lesion and then, using this as a guide, we introduced the TEM rectoscope. After positioning the operative rectoscope, including the optics and surgical instruments, the resection began by marking a 1 cm safety margin around the rectal tumor using high frequency coagulation spots *(Figure 5)* (guided, in case of rectal cancer underwent preoperative radiotherapy, by the previous indian ink marks).

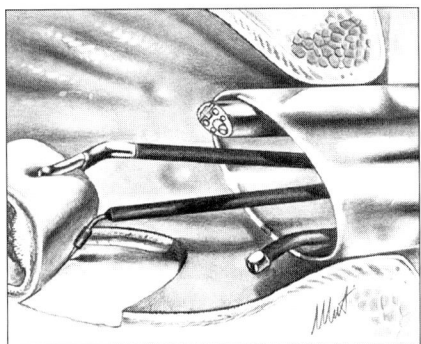

Figure 4. The rectoscope inside the rectum with operative instruments.

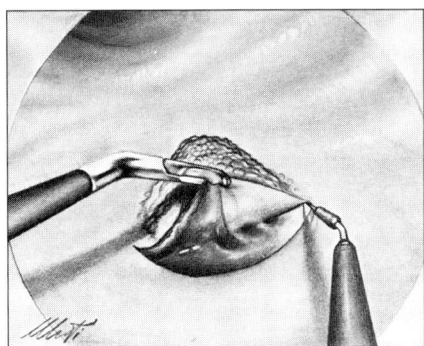

Figure 5. The local excision starting with the electrosurgical knife on the mucosa around the tumor.

Operative options

1. Mucosectomy, removing the mucosa, including the polyp, from the inner circular layer of the muscolaris.

2. Partial wall excision, dividing the circular from the longitudinal muscle layer, for lesions located in the intraperitoneal part of the rectum so as to reduce the risk of a peritoneal breach.

3. Full thickness excision, for lesions located in the extraperitoneal rectum, including perirectal fat and adjacent lymphnodes.

4. Segmental resection, in cases of circumferential tumor growth.

Some authors proposed the ultrasound coagulation to dissect the rectal wall. As previously reported, we consider this technique less precise than the high frequency electrocoagulation and bipolar cutting. Notwithstanding the advantages of the ultrasound coagulation in the dissection of the perirectal vessels (hemorroidary artery), we do not recommend this method because of the damage of the incisional margins around the tumor. Moreover at present only ultrasound straight probes are available with consequent technical problems for a correct transanal endoscopic microsurgical dissection.

In order to prevention cell implantation in malignant tumors, the residual cavity can be irrigated by a Mitomicyn C solution (10 mg diluted in 200 cc of saline) and a povidone iodine solution [5].

The defect was then closed by a running suture of PDS 3.0 monofilament (Ethicon Endo-Surgery, Cincinnati, OH, code number mic160), with a silver clip (Wolf Company, Tuttlingen,Germany) inserted at each end to avoid placing knots in a restricted space *(Figure 6)*.

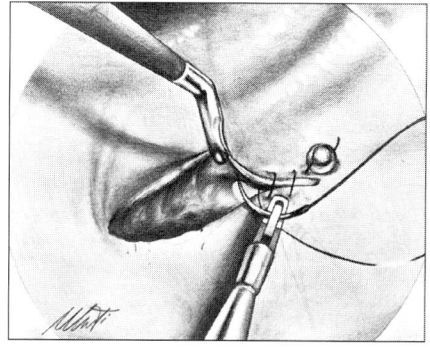

Figure 6. The running suture of the rectal defect with the silver clip positioned at the end of the thread.

Specimen were fixed onto a cork board immediately after resection to measure the extent of the lesion and safety margins.

In patient with rectal cancer, we performed 4-6 macrobiopsies on the proximal and distal verge of the rectum for an intraoperative histological examination in order to determine the completeness of the excision. In such cases, a definitive histological examination determined the grade of the tumor.

In our protocol, each patient was examined 1 and 3 months after being discharged by a clinical examination, a digital rectal exploration and rectoscopy. Succeeding follow-up dates were: for adenomas, after 6 and 12 months, and then, once a year (clinical exploration, rectoscopy with multiple biopsies and endorectal ultrasound); for carcinomas, every 3 months during the first two postoperative years, and then every 6 months (clinical exploration, rectoscopy with multiple biopsies, endorectal ultrasound, MR or CT) [5].

Based on recent literature, **local resection represents an ideal solution for sessile adenomas and it may be also used in selected cases of early rectal cancer** [11-24].

Traditional abdominal and perineal rectal resections are associated with substantial morbidity (20-30%) and mortality (5-10%), particularly for older and high operative risk patients [25].

Tumors in the lower third of the rectum may be resected using a Park retractor but this technique results in poor exposure and can only be used for lesions near the anus [26]. Other approaches are the Mason and Kraske techniques; however, they are more invasive and have higher complication rates (10-15%) [27].

Rectal tumors may also be treated locally by: electrocoagulation [28], endocavitary radiation [29,30], laser vaporization and cryotherapy [31].

One of the most important advantages of Transanal Endoscopic Microsurgery, compared to the other transanal approaches, is the good exposure of the operative field with a **magnified three-dimensional image**, allowing an extremely precise dissection [6].

The position and the angle of the rectoscope within the rectum are crucial to TEM feasibility and permit a wide full thickness excision in large tumors located beyond the valves of the rectal mucosal.

The combination instrument (ICC 350, ERBE Company, Tubingen, Germany) allows rapid switching from the cutting to coagulation mode simply by activing a foot pedal. This combination device, compared with the conventional technique, has the following advantages: a very precise bipolar cutting, an effective monopolar coagulation associated with a continuous suction, a rinsing function allowing the identification of bleeding points. In fact, in cases of bleeding, suction and coagulation are simultaneous and therefore the field visualization is clear, with faster and safer hemostasis [10].

Elective indications for TEM are: sessile rectal adenomas located within 25 cm from the anus and well and moderately well differentiated pT1 carcinomas in the extraperitoneal rectum.

Accurate preoperative staging of these lesions is mandatory and requires a specific diagnostic protocol consisted of clinical examination, endoscopy with multiple macrobiopsies, endorectal ultrasound, and MR and/or CT.

TEM permits the removal of **more invasive rectal tumors** (pT2, pT3) in elderly and high risk patients and in patients who refuse an abdomino-perineal operation. In such cases, is strongly recommended a **preoperative treatment with radiotherapy** [15, 32-34]. In our experience, preoperative radiotherapy did not cause suturing to be more difficult nor did it increase the risk of suture line dehiscence. Leaking suture lines occurred both in radiotherapy and non-radiotherapy patients, without statistically significant differences. Dehiscences occurred only in cases where there was significant tension on the suture line and healed by conservative treatment.

On the other hand, radiotherapy caused a higher tendency for bleeding during dissection, with an increased possibility of occlusion of the suction cannula, resulting in longer operative time.

TEM includes the followings surgical excision techniques: mucosectomy, partial wall excision in the intraperitoneal rectum, to reduce the risk of a peritoneal opening, full thickness excision in the extraperitoneal rectum, segmental resection, in case of circumferential tumor growth.

In our experience, in extraperitoneal lesions, we preferred a full thickness excision also in lesions preoperatively diagnosed as benign because they could have areas of T1 carcinoma. Moreover, when the rectal wall is widely mobilized, as after a full thickness excision, it was easier to perform the suture, with less tension on the margins. In such cases, we preferred full thickness stitches.

A peritoneal breach, which occurs in some cases of resections of large adenomas, can be sutured with double layer stiches by TEM, with no increase of the postoperative complication rate.

The post-TEM complication rate is low, particularly when compared to other surgical techniques, such as low anterior resection or abdomino- perineal resection [35].

One observed complication is dehiscence of the suture line, which occurred in wide full thickness dissections with subsequent tension on the suture line. The suture leak is often partial and heals by conservative treatment and the patients' quality of life is not affected. The clinical outcome of post-TEM suture dehiscence is more favourable than in patients with dehiscence after a low anterior resection. This may be explained by the more limited perirectal fat dissection that takes place with TEM (facilitating a more rapid healing of the dehiscence).

Although the use of TEM in the treatment of T2 and T3 rectal cancers reported herein may be considered anecdotal, our preliminary data indicate a role for TEM associated with other therapeutic options (radio and chemotherapy) in the treatment of more invasive rectal cancer, like pT2 [5]. A multicentric randomized trial concerning preoperative radio-chemotherapy and TEM *versus* traditional surgery started in our institute with cooperation of other centres in Europe and USA; its results will be the subject of subsequent reports.

The advantages of TEM, compared to the other transanal approaches, are: good operative field exposure with a magnified three-dimensional image, (allowing a very precise dissection) minimal postoperative pain, short hospitalization, fast recovery, and absence of skin scars.

The disadvantages of TEM are: the need for precise preoperative tumor staging, special training for the surgeon and the high cost of the instruments.

TEM permits safe, full thickness removal of rectal tumors, with accurate suturing of the defect. In literature, low morbidity and mortality together with a short hospital stay and a rapid return to normal activities were reported.

References

1. Buess G, Mentges B. Transanal Endoscopic Microsurgery (TEM). *Minimally Invasive Terapy* 1992; 1: 101-9.
2. Lezoche E, Guerrieri M, Paganini A, Feliciotti F, Di Pietrantonj F. Is transanal endoscopic microsurgery (TEM) a valid treatment for rectal tumors? *Surg Endosc* 1996; 10: 736-41.

3. Winde G, Nottberg H, Keller R, Schmid KW, Bünte H. Surgical cure for early rectal carcinomas (T1). Transanal Endoscopic Microsurgery vs. Anterior Resection. *Dis Colon Rectum* 1996; 39: 969-76.
4. Heintz A, Morschel M, Junginger T. Comparison of results after transanal endocsopic microsurgery and radical resection for T1 carcinoma of the rectum. *Surg Endosc* 1998; 12: 1145-8.
5. Lezoche E, Guerrieri M, Paganini AM, Feliciotti F. Transanal Endoscopic Microsurgical Excision of irradiated and nonirradiated rectal cancer. A 5 year experience. *Surg Lap & Endosc* 1998; 8: 249-56.
6. Raestrup H, Manncke K, Mentges B, et al. Indications and technique for TEM (Transanal Endoscopic Microsurgery). *Endosc Surg Allied Technol* 1994; 2: 241-6.
7. Sailer M, Leppert R, Kraemer M, Fuchs KH, Thiede A. The value of endorectal ultrasound in the assessment of adenomas, T1- and T2-carcinomas. *Int J Colorectal Dis* 1997; 12: 214-9.
8. Thompson WM, Halvorsen RA, Foster WL Jr. Preoperative and postoperative CT staging of rectosigmoid carcinoma. *Am J Radiol* 1986; 106: 703.
9. Farin G. Pneumatically controlled bipolar cutting instrument. *Endosc Surg Allied Technol* 1993; 1: 97-101.
10. Guerrieri M, Paganini AM, Feliciotti F, Lezoche E. Combination instruments: a report on 95 transanal endoscopic microsurgical operations. *Min Invas Ther & Allied Technol* 1999; 8: 83-7.
11. Kim DG, Madoff RD. Transanal treatment of rectal cancer: ablative methods and open resection. *Semin Surg Oncol* 1998; 15: 101-13.
12. Weber TK, Petrelli NJ. Local excision for rectal cancer: an uncertain future. *Oncology* 1998; 12: 933-43; 944-7.
13. Le Voyer TE, Hoffman JP, Cooper H, Ross E, Sigurdson E, Heisenberg B. Local excision and chemoradiation for low rectal T1 and T2 cancers is an effective treatment. *Am Surg* 1999; 65: 625-30.
14. Minsky BD. Conservative treatment of rectal cancer with local excision and postoperative radiation therapy. *Eur J Cancer* 1995; 31: 1343-6.
15. Rouanet P, Fabre JM, Dubois JB. Conservative surgery for low rectal carcinoma after high-dose radiation. *Ann Surg* 1995; 221: 67-73.
16. Wagman R, Minsky BD, Cohen AM, Saltz L, Paty PB, Guillem JG. Conservative managment of rectal cancer with local excision and postoperative adjuvant therapy. *Int J Radiat Oncol Biol Phys* 1999; 44: 841-6.
17. Chakravarti A, Compton CC, Shellito PC, Wood WC, Landry J, et al. Long-term follow-up of patients with rectal cancers managed by local excision with end without adjuvant irradiation. *Ann Surg* 1999; 239: 49-54.
18. Slisow W, Moesta KT, Schlag PM. Local excision of rectal cancer through windowed specula: long term results. Recent Results. *Cancer Res* 1998; 146: 114-23.
19. Bleday R. Local excision of rectal cancer. *World J Surg* 1997; 21: 706-14.
20. Graham RA, Hackford AW, Wazer DE. Local excision of rectal carcinoma: a safe alternative for more advanced tumors? *J Surg Oncol* 1999; 70: 235-8.
21. Taylor RH, Hay JH, Larsson SN. Transanal local excision of selected low rectal cancers. *Am J Surg* 1998; 175: 360-3.
22. Johnson DE, Hoffman JP. Sphincter preservation in rectal cancer. Surgical considerations for local excision. *Semin Radiat Oncol* 1998; 8: 39-47.
23. Varma MG, Rogers SJ, Schrock TR, Welton ML. Local excision of rectal carcinoma. *Arch Surg* 1999; 134: 863-7.
24. Graham RA, Garnsey L, Jessup JM. Local excision of rectal carcinoma. *Am J Surg* 1990; 160: 306-12.
25. Localio SA, Eng K, Coppa Gf. Abdomino-sacral resection for mid rectal cancer: a fifteen year experience. *Ann Surg* 1983; 198: 320-4.
26. Parks A. A technique for excising extensive villous papillomas in the lower rectum. *Proc R Soc Med* 1968; 1: 101-9.

27. Mason Ay. Surgical access to the rectum: a trans-sphincteric exposure. *Proc R Soc Med* 1970; 63: 91-4.
28. Eisenstat TE, Deck ST, Rubin RJ. Five year survival in patients with carcinoma of the rectum treated by electrocoagulation. *Am J Surg* 1982; 143: 127-30.
29. Hull TL, Lavery TC, Saxon JP. Endocavitary irradiation. An option in select patients with rectal cancer. *Dis Colon Rectum* 1994; 37: 1266-70.
30. Mendenhall WM, Rout WR, Vauthey JN, Haigh LS, Zlotecki RA, Copeland EM 3rd Conservative treatment of rectal adenocarcinoma withendocavitary irradiation or wide local excision and postoperative irradiation. *J Clin Oncol* 1997; 15: 3241-8.
31. Auteri F, Alessandro L. Cryotherapy as an alternative intervention to surgical excision in the management of cancer of the rectum. *Clin Ter* 1993; 142: 347-50.
32. Marks G, Mohiuddin M, Masoni L. The reality of radical sphincter preservation surgery for rectal of the distal 3 cm of rectum following high-dose radiation. *Int J Radiat Oncol Biol Phys* 1993; 27: 779-83.
33. Bozzetti F, Baratti D, Andreola R, Zucari S, Schiavo M, Spinelli P, Gronchi A, Bertario L, Mariani L, Gennari L. Preoperative radiation therapy for patients with T2-T3 carcinoma of the middle-to-lower rectum. *Cancer* 1999; 86: 398-404.
34. Russell AH, Harris J, Rosenberg PJ, Sause WT, Fisher BJ, Hoffman JP, Kraybill WG, Byhardt RW. Anal sphincter conservation for patients with adenocarcinoma of the distal rectum: long-term results of radiation therapy oncology group protocol 89-02. *Int J Radiat Oncol Biol Phys* 2000; 46: 267-8.
35. Willet CG, Compton CC, Shellito PC. Selection factors for local excision or abdominal perineal resection of early stage rectal cancer. *Cancer* 1994; 73: 2716-20.

III

Ultrasound Guided Endoscopic Procedures

Update Gastroenterology 2001.
Tytgat G.N.J., Lundell L., eds. John Libbey Eurotext, Paris © 2001, pp. 63-75.

Endoscopic ultrasound guided fine needle aspiration. A critical appraisal

Peter Vilmann, Jens Thorbøll

Department of Surgical Gastroenterology D, Gentofte University Hospital, Denmark

Endoscopic ultrasound (EUS) is beyond doubt a unique imaging modality with its capability to visualize the gastrointestinal (GI) tract and surrounding organs and structures in great details. Until recently, it was a common believe that EUS imaging alone was able to differentiate benign from malignant lesions in most cases. EUS imaging may assist in the evaluation of the nature of a lesion outlined, but due to false positive diagnoses, suspicious lesions have to be confirmed by tissue evaluation if clinical decisions such as offering major surgery or chemotherapy are made.

Since the first report of direct EUS guided fine needle aspiration (EUS-FNA) was published by our group at Gentofte University Hospital in 1992 [1], the publications on this subject are growing rapidly. EUS-FNA is still a relatively new technique which seems to have an important impact on therapeutic decision-making. A critical evaluation of the outcome of EUS-FNA as well as a definition of its limitations and possible complications are therefore necessary.

The aim of this report is to describe the present status of EUS-FNA based on a literature survey and our personal experiences during more than 10 years and furthermore to outline the possible indications.

Guidelines leading to possible indications for EUS-FNA

The overall sensitivity of EUS-FNA for malignant disease has been reported in the range of 80-85%, with a positive predictive value of 100% (PPV) and an accuracy for all diagnoses between 80-90%. However, the diagnostic values are highly dependent on both the site of the biopsy and the nature of the lesion [2]. Mediastinal tumors and lymph nodes seem to carry the highest diagnostic values with a sensitivity of more than 90% followed by EUS-FNA of pancreatic lesions with a sensitivity between 75-85%. There are also fluctuations in the diagnostic values according to the size of the lesion, but even EUS-FNA of lymph nodes less than 1 cm seems to have a sensibility of around 75% [2, 3]. Endosonography and EUS-FNA are by tradition performed by gastroenterologists. However, the close proximity of the GI tract to organs covered by other specialities makes these organs obvious targets for EUS-FNA. There is no doubt that the role of endosonography has expanded beyond "staging of malignant GI-tumors only" to also include final diagnosis of undiagnosed primary lesions. One of the major indications for EUS-guided biopsy seems to be the evaluation of enlarged lymph nodes suspected of malignancy in the mediastinum or abdomen if not accessible by conventional methods [2-4]. EUS-FNA of lymph nodes has a higher yield and is more reliable than EUS-FNA of extraintestinal masses and GI wall [2]. In a multicenter study with EUS-FNA of 192 lymph nodes in 171 patients, the sensitivity, specificity, PPV, and negative predictive value (NPV) were 93%, 100%, 86%, and 92%, respectively. The sensitivity of EUS-FNA in lymph nodes with a size less than 1 cm (n = 35) was 75% *versus* 96% (n = 157) in lymph nodes more than 1 cm in diameter. Lower cytologic yield was found in another large single center study of 160 lymph nodes [5]. In this study, the sensitivity decreased to 50% *versus* 88% when lymph nodes less than 1 cm compared to more than 1 cm in diameter (n = 17/143) were targeted. As compared with other nodes, cytopuncture of coeliac nodes resulted in greater sensitivity (96% *versus* 82%). It was concluded that EUS-FNA can be considered as a first line technique in the evaluation of unexplained lymphadenopathy. A number of studies have demonstrated that EUS-FNA may be of benefit also for the diagnosis of histoplasmosis [6], sarcoidosis [7, 8], mediastinal tuberculosis [9], Hodgkin lymphoma [10]. In a recent study of 19 patients suspected for sarcoidosis with enlarged lymph nodes located subcarinally, in the aortico-pulmonary window or in the lower posterior mediastinum, EUS-FNA revealed epithelioid cell granulomas suggesting sarcoidosis in all patients [8]. One of these patients was subsequently diagnosed with tuberculosis after a positive mycobacterial culture.

Diagnostic possibilities of EUS-FNA extracted from current publications are listed in *Table I and II*.

EUS-FNA is an interventional procedure and, as all other interventional procedures, a potential risk of complications exists, either from the needle puncture itself or from the manipulation of the endoscope. However, if risky procedures are avoided and basic principles are followed, EUS-FNA is today regarded as a safe procedure [2, 11]. The overall complication rate for solid masses (*e.g.* bleeding, infection, perforation) is less than 1% [11]. Infections following aspiration of cystic lesions occur in up to 14% but may be less if prophylactic antibiotics are given [2, 12].

Minor bleeding is always seen at the puncture side but this is in most cases limited to a few ml [13]. In only a few cases major bleeding necessitating surgery has been described. Perforation, mainly due to manipulation of the endoscope through advanced stenotic tumors, may be seen [2]. Pancreatitis has been described in a few cases related to pancreatic biopsies [14, 15]. These are mainly observations of isolated elevation of s-amylase without symptomatical pancreatitis. Air embolism without any symptomatic consequence has been described in a single case [16]. Tumor cell seeding after EUS-FNA, although never

Table I. Primary diagnoses that may be obtained by EUS-FNA

Location	Type of lesion	Diagnosis
Mediastinum	Primary tumors	– Esophageal cancer – Submucosal tumors of the esophagus, leiomyoma and leio-myosarcoma or other stromal tumors, lymphoma, foregut-cysts – Lung cancer and mesothelioma – Thymoma, schwannoma, spindle cell tumor, malignant histiocytoma, sarcoma, teratoma, thymoma, neuroendocrine tumor and mediastinal stroma
Mediastinum	Lymph nodes	– Metastases from undiagnosed primary tumors: breast cancer, gynecological cancer, GI cancer, lung cancer and miscellaneous cancers such as melanoma – Lymphoma – Sarcoidosis – Histoplasmosis – Tuberculosis
Abdomen	Primary and secondary tumors	– Gastric and duodenal tumors: carcinomas, submucosal stromal tumors and lymphomas – Pancreatic tumors: carcinomas, neuroendocrine tumors, secondary tumors – Primary hepatobiliary tumors: hepatocellular carcinomas and biliary carcinomas – Liver metastases – Submucosal tumors of the rectum – Miscellaneous: primary and secondary tumors of the adrenal glands, the prostate and seminal vesicles
Abdomen	Lymph nodes	– Metastases from undiagnosed primary tumors: breast cancer, gynecologic cancer, GI cancer, lung cancer, prostatic cancer and miscellaneous cancers – Lymphomas – Miscellaneous: sarcoidosis, tuberculosis

Table II. Cancers where EUS-FNA may have an important role in the staging prior to therapy

Location	Lymph nodes or metastases to organs	Diagnosis
Mediastinum	Staging	– Lung cancer – GI cancer: esophageal cancer, gastric cancer, pancreatic cancer – Lymphomas – Miscellaneous: gynecological cancer, urological cancer, breast cancer
Abdomen	Staging	– Esophageal cancer – Gastric and duodenal cancer – Pancreatic cancer and malignant neuroendocrine tumors – Hepatobiliary cancer – Lymphomas – Miscellaneous: urological cancer, gynecological cancer, breast cancer

published, is a potential problem which has created some concern. However, as judged from results obtained from large studies with transcutaneous ultrasound guided FNA, tumor cell seeding seems to be a very limited problem. Avoidance of biopsy through tumor infiltrated wall layers should always be respected. A theoretical advantage of EUS-FNA compared to transcutaneous biopsy is the short needle tract. Moreover, this needle tract will in most cases be resected obviating the risk of spreading malignant cells distant from the main lesion. An example of this is biopsy of malignant pancreatic lesions with subsequent Whipple's resection.

Esophageal carcinoma

The indications of EUS-FNA of lymph nodes in patients with esophageal cancer is dependent on the therapeutic strategy. It is generally agreed that there are no indications for EUS-FNA of local lymph nodes unless the patients are offered stage-dependent chemo/radiation therapy, whereas EUS-FNA of lymph nodes regarded as distant metastases seems to have a higher impact on the therapeutic decisions [17]. A few studies have addressed the role of EUS-FNA regarding diagnosis of lymph node involvement in esophageal cancer [17-19]. A study from France has retrospectively evaluated the impact of EUS-FNA in 40 patients out of 198 (20%) with suspected distant lymph node metastases and esophageal cancer [17]. Among these, 19 had cervical lymph nodes, 10 mediastinal and 11 patients had coeliac lymph nodes. Malignant cells were found in 31 cases and benign cells in 8 cases with one technical failure. The diagnosis obtained by EUS-FNA led to a change in management in 60% of the patients. In another study of 62 patients considered resectable by CT scan, 17 patients had lymph nodes suspected of malignancy located at the coeliac axis [18]. In 15 patients, distant lymph node metastases were confirmed by EUS-FNA. In addition, EUS-FNA seems valuable also for evaluation of lymph nodes after therapy and possible down-staging effect of radio/chemotherapy [17, 19]. Further studies are needed before firm conclusions may be drawn regarding the role of EUS-FNA for staging of lymph nodes in esophageal cancer.

Mediastinal tumors and lung cancer

EUS gives an outstanding view over the posterior mediastinum, including the subcarinal region, the inferior mediastinum and the aorticopulmonary window. However, EUS is of limited value in the pretracheal and partly in the paratracheal region. An increasing number of papers describe the use of EUS-FNA in the evaluation of mediastinal pathology. Publications on EUS-FNA of primary mediastinal lesions outlined by CT scan and subsequently diagnosed by EUS-FNA include, among others, lung cancer, mesothelioma, schwannoma, lymphoma, spindle cell tumor, malignant histiocytoma, sarcoma, teratoma, thymoma, mediastinal struma and neuro-endocrine tumor [20-28].

Several studies have shown that EUS-FNA is valuable for primary diagnosis of suspected lung cancer. This was demonstrated in a study with 9 patients referred for EUS-FNA with mediastinal masses on CT [2]. All 6 patients with a final diagnosis of lung cancer were diagnosed either as having non-small-cell lung cancer (NSCLC) or small-cell lung cancer (SCLC) by EUS-FNA. Another study of 35 patients with suspected lung cancer in whom bronchoscopic methods failed showed EUS-FNA to be highly accurate for the diagnosis of lung cancer when lymph nodes were targeted [29]. In 25 patients, malignancy was confirmed by EUS-FNA, 11 adenocarcinomas, 10 SCLC, 3 squamous cell carcinomas and 1 lymphoma. The sensitivity, specificity and accuracy were 96%, 100% and 97 respectively. In 7 patients, the punctured nodes were less than 1 cm in diameter, which are difficult to sample by other methods.

In addition to this, EUS-FNA have been evaluated also for staging of NSCLC, either in retrospective designs or prospectively in comparison with CT and/or mediastinoscopy [28-32]. One of these studies demonstrated an accuracy of 96% regarding EUS-FNA of mediastinal nodes in the preoperative evaluation of 24 patients with known NSCLC mediastinoscopy [28] compared to 49% accuracy of the CT scan. The result of EUS-FNA prompted a change in management in 95% of the patients undergoing EUS-FNA. Another study compared EUS-FNA with mediastinoscopy and reported a sensitivity of 100% and 86%, respectively with a 100% specificity of both the procedures [30]. The role of EUS-FNA for staging of NSCLC seems to be complementary to mediastinoscopy and there is some evidence that EUS-FNA should precede mediastinoscopy in patients with CT positive lymph nodes in stations accessible to EUS-FNA [33]. This strategy is strongly supported by a cost-effective study comparing EUS-FNA with mediastinoscopy in patients with NSCLC. The cost-effective advantage conferred by EUS-FNA remained even down to a NPV value of EUS-FNA of 22% [33]. Whether EUS-FNA staging of lymph nodes is of benefit in unselected lung cancer patients is still unknown. Further studies should focus on this, as well as on a prospective controlled and blinded comparison with other staging modalities such as CT, mediastinoscopy, transbronchial biopsy and positron emission tomography scanning.

Submucosal tumors

EUS-guided biopsy of lesions within the GI wall has the lowest diagnostic value and the highest rate of inconclusive biopsies as compared to biopsy of extra-luminal lesions [2, 25]. In a large multicenter study, 115 lesions were located within the GI wall [2]. The accuracy of EUS-FNA of 12 submucosal tumors was 50%, with one half of the biopsy specimens being inadequate. In cases of smooth muscle tumors, although cytology demonstrated spindle cells in four of seven cases, the single case of a leiomyosarcoma was not diagnosed.

In contrast to this, a Japanese study of 22 submucosal tumors concluded that EUS-FNA seems valuable for diagnosis of submucosal tumors [34]. The diagnostic values in this study were superior to the Western experience with a sensitivity, specificity and accuracy of 75%, 100% and 95% respectively. However, only 3 of 4 malignant tumors were diagnosed and insufficient material was experienced in additional 4 patients.

EUS-FNA of submucosal pathology excluding stromal tumors seems to be more successful. In the multicenter study of Wiersema [2], EUS-FNA was performed in 103 lesions arising in the GI wall, exclusive of stromal tumors with a sensitivity, specificity, positive predictive value, negative predictive value, and accuracy of 61%, 79%, 100%, 76%, and 67%, respectively.

The indications for EUS-FNA of submucosal tumors seems less obvious and further studies are needed.

Gastric carcinoma

The role of EUS-FNA for lymph node staging of gastric cancer is not well addressed. Unless stage-dependent chemotherapy is considered prior to surgery, there is no indication for EUS-FNA of local lymph nodes suspected for malignancy in patients with gastric cancer. A few publications with a large number of biopsies from a variety of lesions seem to include patients with gastric cancer for EUS-FNA with suspicious distant lymph node metastases [2, 3, 25, 35]. Further studies are needed to evaluate the role of EUS-FNA in gastric cancer.

Gastric lymphoma

The role of EUS-FNA in patients suspected of gastric lymphoma is not well validated. However, it may be possible to establish the diagnosis by EUS guided fine needle cytology [2]. In this-multi center study, 8 out of 9 gastric non-Hodgkin lymphomas were correctly diagnosed by EUS-FNA. Flow cytometry and immunocytochemistry of cytological specimens obtained by EUS-FNA seem to be advantageous in this evaluation [36]. This study demonstrated an increase in sensitivity from 44% to 86% by using these methods. Further studies are needed before conclusions may be drawn regarding the role of EUS in gastric lymphoma.

Upper gastrointestinal wall thickening

A few studies have addressed the role of EUS in the diagnostic approach to large gastric folds. EUS has a nearby 100% specificity but a lower sensitivity for malignancy. EUS-FNA may occasionally be of benefit if conventional methods fail with a sensitivity of around 60% [2]. However, EUS-FNA failed to diagnose 15 of 25 gastric adenocarcinomas in this study (sensitivity 40%). Further studies and possible improvement regarding EUS-FNA should be encouraged.

Pancreatic carcinoma

Due to the limitations of EUS imaging to differentiate between malignant and inflammatory pancreatic lesions as well as surrounding lymph nodes, a considerable interest in EUS-FNA exists. Several publications have demonstrated that EUS-FNA of focal pancreatic tumors is possible with a reported sensitivity for malignant disease in the range from 68% to 96% [2, 15, 37-44]. There exists no prospective blinded studies between EUS-FNA and CT or US transcutaneous guided biopsy. The main problem of EUS-FNA of the pancreas is a relatively low NPV which means that a negative biopsy cannot rule out malignancy. A high rate of insufficient biopsies are seen from 5% to 20%, highest in centers without a cytopathologist immediately available to confirm the sufficiency of the aspirate [2, 45]. A study from the USA reported that 5 to 6 needle passes should be made for pancreatric masses when a cytopathologist is not in attendance [2, 46]. The only factor that predicted the number of FNAs required in order to make a diagnosis was the differentiation of the tumor.

However, it seems that EUS-FNA has a major impact on therapeutic decisions and especially in those cases where other imaging techniques are incapable of visualizing the lesion [39, 47]. This is the case by CT in up to 20-40%, mainly when tumors are less than 2-3 cm in diameter. A change in management when EUS-FNA is performed is reported to be as high as 60%, either by confirmation of malignancy, diagnosis of neuroendocrine tumors or secondary pancreatic neoplasms, diagnosis of surrounding lymph node metastases or distant metastases in the liver excluding curative therapy [39, 48]. A multicenter study included 124 patients with pancreatic lesions. The diagnostic values for pancreatic masses demonstrated a sensitivity of 86%, a specificity of 94%, a PPV of 100%, an NPV of 86%, and an accuracy of 88% [2]. These diagnostic values were obtained with a median number of needle passes of 2 (range 1-19). Another large single center study with 144 patients found a sensitivity of 72% with a NPV of 38% [25]. If atypical cytology was considered diagnostic for malignancy, the sensitivity and NPV changed to 82% and 51%, respectively. There was no difference in diagnostic values when stratified by size, either more than 3 cm or less than 3 cm.

A study from Texas, USA, demonstrated in contrast a very high sensitivity of 96% in 98 patients [42]. In 21% no mass was seen by CT in this study. Another study from France with 99 patients demonstrated a low overall diagnostic yield of 68%, a sensitivity of 75%, an accuracy of 68% and a NPV of 37% [43].

The role for EUS-FNA in the assessment of lymph nodes in patients with pancreatic cancer can be extracted from a few studies and it seems that lymphatic spread may be confirmed in a considerable number of patients [38, 39, 42, 47]. In a study from Texas, USA, with 98 patients with pancreatic lesions, lymph nodes were targeted in 27 patients [42]. EUS-FNA determined that 18 patients (32% of patients with adenocarcinoma) had positive lymph nodes. However, prospective studies with EUS-FNA in comparison with surgical findings should be made before the exact role of EUS-FNA in the evaluation of lymph node metastases in patients with pancreatic cancer may be found. More studies comparing different modalities are needed in the evaluation of EUS-FNA in respect to pancreatic carcinoma before firm conclusions may be drawn.

Islet cell neoplasms

The role of EUS-FNA for the diagnosis of islet cell neoplasms is not well validated although confirmative diagnoses have been obtained by this method in a number of cases [2, 25, 42, 43, 49]. The diagnoses include neuroendocrine tumors such as insulinoma and gastrinoma located in the pancreas.

Ampullary carcinoma

The role of EUS-FNA in patients with ampulary carcinomas has never been addressed. In advanced ampullary carcinomas, EUS-FNA may play a role for primary diagnosis if conventional methods such as endoscopic mucosal biopsy fail but these cases are usually indistinguishable from primary pancreatic cancers [42].

Gallbladder and bile ducts

One study from Germany has reported EUS-FNA to have a potential role for diagnosis of hilar cholangiocarcinoma, especially when standard methods are inconclusive [50]. In this study, 10 patients with bile duct strictures at the hepatic hilum diagnosed by CT and/or ERCP underwent EUS-FNA. In 9 patients with an adequate aspirate, cholangiocarcinoma was diagnosed in 7 patients and hepatocellular carcinoma in one patient. EUS-FNA was false negative in the last patient. Further studies are needed.

Liver

EUS has not been used extensively in imaging the liver. Although portions of the left lobe are imaged from the stomach and part of the right lobe from the stomach and duodenum, inadequate penetration prevents imaging of the entire liver. Transcutaneous ultrasound and CT provide a more complete examination of the liver than does EUS, although no prospective comparisons of these modalities in the detection of focal liver abnormalities are available. A few retrospective studies have reported EUS-FNA to be able to diagnose small liver lesions not detected by CT or transcutaneous US [2, 51, 52]. In a case study, a small recurrent hepatocellular carcinoma was diagnosed by EUS-FNA in spite of negative US and CT [51]. A multi-center study of 457 patients included 12 selected patients with liver lesions. EUS-FNA was positive for cancer in 100% [2]. In another retrospective study with 14 patients having 15 liver lesions with a median diameter of 1.1 cm, EUS-FNA diagnosed malignant cells in 14 and benign cells in one [52]. Before EUS, CT depicted liver lesions in only 3 of 14 patients (21%). Seven of 14 patients had a known cancer diagnosis. For the other 7, the initial diagnosis of cancer was made by means of EUS-FNA of the liver. In a study with 110 pancreatic EUS-FNAs, 8 patients underwent aspiration of 8 liver metastases, all of which were cytologically positive [46]. Further studies are needed before the exact role of EUS-FNA in the diagnosis of liver lesions is found.

Miscellaneous

A few publications have presented cases in which EUS-FNA was able to diagnose primary or secondary lesions in the left adrenal gland [53]. Before EUS-FNA is performed, pheochromocytoma should be ruled out due to a potential risk of severe hypertension. Also diagnosis of fluid collections can be made by EUS-FNA [54]. If ascites or pleural effusions are seen during an EUS examination in a patient with cancer, carcinosis should be suspected. Frequently, small fluid collections not recognized by other imaging modalities are seen. If malignant cells are seen in the fluid, carcinosis is verified and the patient is not considered for surgical resection. Further studies are needed.

Rectal carcinoma

Only a few case reports on EUS-FNA for diagnosis of rectal carcinoma have been published [55, 56] including one patient with secondary rectal linitis plastica in whom endoscopic biopsies were negative and 2 patients with recurrent rectal cancer in a colorectal anastomosis, all of which were positive by EUS-FNA. Others have shown a high diagnostic yield for diagnosis of perirectal malignancy also in patients with rectal cancer [25]. A multicenter study included 9 patients with perirectal masses demonstrating a sensitivity of EUS-FNA of 100% [2].

Large prospective studies comparing EUS-FNA of perirectal lymph nodes in patients with rectal cancer with surgical pathology are awaited.

Suggestions to indications for EUS-FNA

EUS-FNA seems reasonable in patients with lesions suspicious for malignancy on conventional imaging modalities when standard approaches to tissue diagnosis are unsuccessful or risky [2, 45]. Also, lesions suggestive of malignancy that are detected only by EUS and not by conventional modalities may be biopsied if an aspirate positive for malignancy may change patient management.

Although final indications for EUS-FNA are not fully found at present, possible directions seems possible to extract from a review of the present literature and our own experience with EUS-FNA and suggested as follows:

1. Diagnosis of primary mediastinal tumors if not obtained by conventional methods.

2. Diagnosis of lung cancer or mesothelioma visualized by CT or MRI, located adjacent to the esophagus and not diagnosed by conventional biopsy methods.

3. Confirmation of lung cancer invasion of the mediastinum if suspected by CT (stage T-4).

4. Lymph node staging in patients with malignant tumors if clinically relevant before therapeutic intervention in patients with lung cancer, esophageal cancer, gastric cancer, pancreatic cancer or rectal cancer.

5. Lymph node staging in cancer patients after radio-chemo-therapy if lymph nodes are detected by other imaging modalities and clinically relevant.

6. Lymph node staging in a variety of cancers such as gynecological cancer or urological cancer if enlarged lymph nodes are detected by other imaging techniques but not accessible by conventional methods.

7. Diagnosis of primary mucosal or submucosal tumors not diagnosed by conventional methods.

8. Diagnosis of local submucosal cancer recurrence (esophageal, gastric and rectal cancer).

9. Diagnosis of lymph node enlargement visualized by other imaging techniques, such as CT, US or MR if undiagnosed by conventional methods.

10. Diagnosis of pancreatic lesions suspicious of malignancy and not visible by conventional methods or undiagnosed by CT or US guided biopsy.

11. Diagnosis of neuroendocrine tumors of the pancreas not diagnosed by conventional methods.

12. Diagnosis of tumors in organs adjacent to the GI tract not finally diagnosed by conventional methods, *i.e.* adrenal glands, the liver, the prostate and the lower genito-urinary tract.

13. Diagnosis of fluid collections in patients with suspicion of ascitogenic carcinomatosis, malignant pleural effusion or malignant cysts if outlined during EUS.

References

1. Vilmann P, Hancke S, Henriksen FW, Jacobsen GK. Endoscopic ultrasonography with guided fine needle aspiration biopsy in pancreatic disease. A new diagnostic procedure. *Gastrointest Endosc* 1992; 38: 172-3.
2. Wiersema MJ, Vilmann P, Giovannini M, *et al.* Endosonography guided fine needle aspiration biopsy: diagnostic accuracy and complication assessment. *Gastroenterology* 1997; 112: 1087-95.
3. Vilmann P. Endoscopic ultrasonography-guided fine needle aspiration biopsy of lymph nodes. *Gastrointest Endosc* 1996; 43: S24.
4. Bhutani MS, Hawes RH, Hoffman BJ. A comparison of the accuracy of echo features during endoscopic ultrasound (EUS) and EUS-guided fine-needle aspiration for diagnosis of malignant lymph node invasion. *Gastrointest Endosc* 1997; 45: 474-9.
5. Williams DB, Sahai AV, Aabakken L, *et al.* Endoscopic ultrasound guided fine needle aspiration biopsy: a large single centre experience. *Gut* 1999; 44: 720-6.

6. Wiersema MJ, Chak A, Wiersema LM. Mediastinal histoplasmosis: evaluation with endosonography and endoscopic fine-needle aspiration biopsy. *Gastrointest Endosc* 1994; 40: 78-81.
7. Mishra G, Sahai AV, Penman ID, et al. Endoscopic ultrasonography with fine-needle aspiration: an accurate and simple diagnostic modality for sarcoidosis. *Endoscopy* 1999; 31: 377-82.
8. Fritscher-Ravens A, Sriram PVJ, Topalidis T, et al. Diagnosing sarcoidosis using endosonography-guided fine needle aspiration. *Chest* 2000; 118: 928-35.
9. Kochhar R, Sriram PV, Rajwanshi A, et al. Transesophageal endoscopic fine-needle aspiration cytology in mediastinal tuberculosis. *Gastrointest Endosc* 1999; 50: 271-4.
10. Lewis JD, Faigel DO, Dowdy Y, et al. Hodgkin's disease diagnosed by endoscopic ultrasound-guided fine needle aspiration of a periduodenal lymph node. *Am J Gastroenterol* 1998; 93: 834.
11. Vilmann P, Hancke S. A new biopsy handle instrument for endoscopic ultrasound-guided fine-needle aspiration biopsy. *Gastrointest Endosc* 1996; 43: 238-42.
12. O'Toole D, Palazzo L, Arotcarena R, Dancour A, Aubert A, Hammel P, Amaris J, Ruszniewski P. Assessment of complications of EUS-guided fine-needle aspiration. *Gastrointest Endosc* 2001; 53: 470-4.
13. Affi A, Vazquez-Sequeiros E, Norton ID, et al. Acute extraluminal hemorrhage associated with EUS-guided fine needle aspiration: frequency and clinical significance. *Gastrointest Endosc* 2001; 53: 221-5.
14. Gress FG, Hawes RH, Savides TJ, et al. Endoscopic ultrasound-guided fine-needle aspiration biopsy using linear array and radial scanning endosonography. *Gastrointest Endosc* 1997; 45: 243-50.
15. Binmoeller KF, Thul R, Rathod V, et al. Endoscopic ultrasound-guided, 18-gauge, fine needle aspiration biopsy of the pancreas using a 2.8 mm channel array echoendoscope. *Gastrointest Endosc* 1998; 47: 121-7.
16. Pfaffenbach B, Wegener M, Bohmeke T. Hepatic portal venous gas after transgastric EUS-guided fine-needle aspiration of an accessory spleen. *Gastrointest Endosc* 1996; 5: 515-8.
17. Giovannini M, Monges G, Seitz JF, et al. Distant lymph node metastases in esophageal cancer: impact of endoscopic ultrasound-guided biopsy. *Endoscopy* 1999; 31: 536-40.
18. Reed CE, Mishra G, Sahai AV, et al. Esophageal cancer staging: improved accuracy by endoscopic ultrasound of celiac lymph nodes. *Ann Thorac Surg* 1999; 67: 319-21.
19. Penman ID, Williams DB, Sahai AV, et al. Ability of EUS with fine-needle aspiration to document nodal staging and response to neoadjuvant chemoradiotherapy in locally advanced esophageal cancer: a case report. *Gastrointest Endosc* 1999; 49: 783-6.
20. Pedersen BH, Vilmann P, Milman N, et al. Endoscopic ultrasonography with guided fine needle aspiration biopsy of a mediastinal mass lesion. *Acta Radiol* 1995; 36: 326-8.
21. Pedersen BH, Vilmann P, Folke K, et al. Endoscopic ultrasonography and realtime guided fine-needle aspiration biopsy of solid lesions of the mediastinum suspected of malignancy. *Chest* 1996; 110: 539-44.
22. Wiersema MJ, Vilmann P, Giovannini M, et al. Endosonography guided fine needle aspiration biopsy: diagnostic accuracy and complication assessment. *Gastroenterology* 1997; 112: 1087-95.
23. Le Dreau G, Calament G, Volant A, et al. Diagnosis of neuroendocrine tumor of the mediastinum by endosonography guided fine needle aspiration biopsy. *Gastroenterol Clin Biol* 1998; 22: 87-90.
24. Hünerbein M, Ghadimi BM, Haensch W, Schlag PM. Transesophageal biopsy of mediastinal and pulmonary tumors by means of endoscopic ultrasound guidance. *J Thorac Cardiovasc Surg* 1998; 116: 554-9.
25. Williams DB, Sahai AV, Aabakken L, et al. Endoscopic ultrasound guided fine needle aspiration biopsy: a large single centre experience. *Gut* 1999; 44: 720-6.
26. Fritscher-Ravens A, Soehendra N, Schirrow L, et al. Role of transesophageal endosonography-guided fine needle aspiration in the diagnosis of lung cancer. *Chest* 2000; 117: 339-45.
27. McGrath KM, Ballo MS, Jowell PS. Schwannoma of the mediastinum diagnosed by EUS-guided fine needle aspiration. *Gastrointest Endosc* 2001; 53: 362-5.

28. Gress FG, Savides TJ, Sandler A, et al. Endoscopic ultrasonography, fine-needle aspiration biopsy guided by endoscopic ultrasonography, and computed tomography in the preoperative staging of non-small-cell lung cancer: a comparison study. *Ann Intern Med* 1997; 127: 604-12.
29. Fritscher-Ravens A, Sriram PVJ, Bobrowski C, et al. Mediastinal lymphadenopathy in patients with or without previous malignancy: EUS-FNA-based differential cytodiagnosis in 153 patients. *Am J Gastroenterol* 2000; 95: 2278-84.
30. Serna DL, Aryan HE, Chang KJ, et al. An early comparison between endoscopic ultrasound-guided fine-needle aspiration and mediastinoscopy for diagnosis of mediastinal malignancy. *Am Surg* 1998; 64: 1014-8.
31. Silvestri GA, Hoffman BJ, Bhutani MS, et al. Endoscopic ultrasound with fine-needle aspiration in the diagnosis and staging of lung cancer. *Ann Thorac Surg* 1996; 61: 1441-5.
32. Wiersema MJ, Vazques-Sequeiros E, Wiersema LM. Evaluation of mediastinal lymphadenopathy with endoscopic US-guided fine needle aspiration biopsy. *Radiol* 2001; 219: 252-7.
33. Aabakken L, Silvestri GA, Hawes R, et al. Cost-efficacy of Endoscopic ultrasonography with fine-needle aspiration *vs* mediastinoscopy in patients with lung cancer and suspected mediastinal adenopathy. *Endoscopy* 1999; 31: 707-11.
34. Matsui M, Goto H, Niwa Y, et al. Preliminary results of fine needle aspiration biopsy histology in upper gastrointestinal submucosal tumors. *Endoscopy* 1998; 30: 750-5.
35. Hünerbein M, Dohmoto M, Rau B, et al. Endosonography and endosonography-guided biopsy of upper-GI-tract tumors using a curved-array echoendoscope. *Surg Endosc* 1996; 10: 1205-9.
36. Ribeiro A, Vazquez-Sequeiros E, Wiersema LM, Wang KK, Clain JE, Wiersema MJ. EUS-guided fine-needle aspiration combined with flow cytometri and immunocytochemistry in the diagnosis of lymphoma. *Gastrointest Endosc* 2001; 53: 485-91.
37. Vilmann P, Giovannini M, Siemsen M, Wiersema M. EUS-guided biopsy of pancreatic lesions suspected of malignancy: a multicentre study. *Acta Endoscopica* 1995; 25: 465.
38. Cahn M, Chang K, Nguyen P, Butler J. Impact of endoscopic ultrasound with fine-needle aspiration on the surgical management of pancreatic cancer. *Am J Surg* 1996; 172: 470-2.
39. Chang KJ, Nguyen P, Erickson RA, et al. The clinical utility of endoscopic ultrasound-guided fine-needle aspiration in the diagnosis and staging of pancreatic carcinoma. *Gastrointest Endosc* 1997; 45: 387-9.
40. Bhutani MS, Hawes RH, Baron PL, et al. Endoscopic ultrasound guided fien needle aspiration of malignant pancreatic lesions. *Endoscopy* 1997; 29: 854-8.
41. Faigel DO, Ginsberg GG, Bentz JS, et al. Endoscopic ultrasound-guided real-time fine-needle aspiration biopsy of the pancreas in cancer patients with pancreatic lesions. *J Clin Oncol* 1997;15: 1439-43.
42. Suits J, Frazee R, Erickson RA. Endoscopic ultrasound and fine needle aspiration for the evaluation of pancreatic masses. *Arch Surg* 1999; 134: 639-42.
43. Voss M, Hammel P, Molas G, et al. Value of endoscopic ultrasound guided fine needle aspiration biopsy in the diagnosis of solid pancreatic masses. *Gut* 2000; 46: 244-9.
44. Fritscher-Ravens A, Izbicki JR, Sriram PV, et al. Endosonography-guided, fine-needle aspiration cytology extending the indications for organ-preserving pancreatic surgery. *Am J Gastroenterol* 2000; 95: 2255-60.
45. Chang KJ, Katz KD, Durbin TE, et al. Endoscopic ultrasound-guided fine needle aspiration. *Gastrointest Endosc* 1994; 40: 694-6.
46. Erickson RA, Sayage-Rabie L, Beissner S. Factors predicting the number of EUS-guided fine-needle passes for diagnosis of pancreatic malignancies. *Gastrointest Endosc* 2000; 51: 184-90.
47. Erickson RA, Garza AA. Impact of endoscopic ultrasound on the management and outcome of pancreatic carcinoma. *Am J Gastroenterol* 2000; 95: 2248-54.
48. Frazee RC, Singh H, Erickson RA. Endoscopic ultrasound for peripancreatic masses. *Am J Surg* 1997; 174: 596-8.

49. Kirkeby H, Vilmann P, Burcharth F. Insulinoma diagnosed by endoscopic ultrasonography guided biopsy. J. Laparoendosc. *Adv Surg Tech A* 1999; 9: 295-8.
50. Fritscher-Ravens A, Broering DC, Sriram PV, et al. EUS-guided fine-needle aspiration cytodiagnosis of hilar cholangiocarcinoma: a case series. *Gastrointest Endosc* 2000; 52: 534-40.
51. Bogstad J, Vilmann P, Burchardt F. Early detection of recurrent hepatocellular carcinoma by endosonographically guided fine-needle aspiration biopsy. *Endoscopy* 1997; 29: 322-4.
52. Nguyen P, Feng JC, Chang KJ. Endoscopic ultrasound (EUS) and EUS-guided fine needle aspiration of liver lesions. *Gastrointest Endosc* 1999; 50: 357-61.
53. Chang KJ, Erickson RA, Nguyen P. Endoscopic ultrasound (EUS) and EUS guided fine-needle aspiration of the left adrenal gland. *Gastrointest Endosc* 1996; 44:568-71.
54. Chang KJ, Albers CG, Nguyen P. Endoscopic ultrasound-guided fine needle aspiration of pleural and ascitic fluid. *Am J Gastroenterol* 1995; 90: 148-50.
55. Bhutani MS. EUS and EUS-guided fine-needle aspiration for the diagnosis of rectal linitis plastica secondary to prostate carcinoma. *Gastrointest Endosc* 1999; 50: 117-9.
56. Woodward T, Menke D. Diagnosis of recurrent rectal carcinoma by EUS-guided fine-needle aspiration. *Gastrointest Endosc* 2000; 51: 223-5.

EUS-guided celiac plexus neurolysis

Paul Fockens

Department of Gastroenterology, Academic Medical Center, University of Amsterdam, Amsterdam, Netherlands

Management of pancreatic pain is difficult. Especially in pancreatic cancer, pain may be difficult to treat with medication and for this reason celiac plexus neurolysis (CPN) was developed early last century [1]. The aim of CPN is to chemically destruct the ganglia around the celiac trunc. Although developed as a surgical technique during laparotomy, other less invasive methods have been developed. In order to improve the accuracy of delivery and thereby the results, radiological guidance was introduced. Initially fluoroscopy was used but later CT-guided CPN became more popular. There are different ways to approach the celiac plexus, posterior or anterior, and many adjustments were made to the technique including even posterior trans-aortic CPN.

Endoscopic ultrasonography (EUS) was introduced in the early eighties as a high-resolution diagnostic imaging technique. EUS proved to have a high accuracy for pancreatic cancer staging, with results between 85% and 95% [2]. After introduction of curved linear array echoendoscopes, EUS-guided fine needle aspiration biopsies became possible in the early nineties. This addition to the armamentarium of the echoendoscopist allowed for low-risk, high-accuracy cytological diagnosis of extraluminal lesions such as pancreatic tumors and/or lymph nodes. The technique has been extensively evaluated and has been shown to be highly accurate and to have very few complications [3].

In 1996, the first publication on EUS-guided CPN appeared in literature, using the same technique and instruments as that of EUS-guided biopsies [4]. Nowadays the more invasive part of EUS is called interventional EUS and EUS-guided CPN is only one of its rapidly increasing number of indications.

Technique

Patient preparation consists of nil by mouth for 6 hours or more and blood test for normal coagulation parameters. Some authors have described routine pre-hydration with 200-500 ml of normal saline. Patients are placed in left decubitus position and sedated with midazolam which can be combined with a morfinomimetic drug. A curved linear array echoendoscope is always the instrument of choice, such as manufactured by Olympus, Pentax or Toshiba. The diameter of the channel can be standard or larger. A standard 22 or 23 Gauge needle such as also used for fine-needle-aspiration biopsies is used. Although the newer echoendoscopes are equipped with video-endoscopy, there is no need for this in this procedure as it is entirely performed under EUS-guidance. Similarly a balloon sheath around the transducer is not necessary for this indication.

After introduction of the echoendoscope in the esophagus, localization of the celiac trunk is straightforward. In the esophagus the descending aorta is identified by rotating the instrument and after that the aorta is followed caudally. The crus of the diaphragm is seen just cranial to the origin of the celiac trunk and superior mesenteric artery. These vessels are usually seen in the same image between 40 and 45 cm from the incisors. The ganglia of the celiac plexus are not identified as a discrete structure on EUS but they are located just to the right and left side of the origin of the celiac trunk.

One can choose between two types of injection, either two injections on both sides of the origin of the celiac trunk or one combined injection just cranially of the trunk. The rapid dissolution of the fluid in the loose retroperitoneal tissue will allow equal spreading to both sides. Here we will only describe the single injection technique in more detail. After the needle has been advanced into the area just above the origin of the celiac trunk, the needle is flushed with 2 ml of normal saline and an aspiration test is performed to assure the tip of the needle is not in a vessel. After this aspiration test, 6-8 ml of a local anesthetic agent is injected (Bupivacaine 0.25%). The aspiration test is repeated and then a total of 20 ml absolute (98%) alcohol is injected. During injection an echo-rich cloud is typically seen on EUS. The needle is then again flushed with some saline before withdrawal from the endoscope and removal of the echoendoscope from the patient. Patients are observed for a minimum of two hours with special attention for orthostatic complaints that may occasionally occur.

Indications and results

The indications for EUS-guided CPN are not different from the techniques of celiac plexus neurolysis. Patients with pain from an irresectable pancreatic cancer are probably the best candidates for this treatment. In a large surgical study published in 1993, CPN during surgery was compared to placebo in patients who were explored for pancreatic cancer and proved to be irresectable [5]. In this study, patients received celiac plexus neurolysis with ethanol or placebo, and were stratified to whether or not they had pain prior to exploration. Patients in the ethanol treated group (both with pain and also those without preoperative pain) had lower pain scores during the 6-month follow-up than the placebo group.

Furthermore a survival benefit was found for those patients with preoperative pain treated with ethanol compared to the placebo group.

The largest series of EUS-guided CPN was recently published in Gastrointestinal Endoscopy [6]. The authors describe their experience from 1995 to 1998 in 58 patients undergoing EUS-guided CPN for pain from an irresectable pancreatic cancer. The authors used one EUS-procedure in most patients to obtain a cytological diagnosis, to stage the patients and to treat their pain complaints with EUS-guided CPN. This combined use of different EUS-techniques during one investigation provides optimal patient care and maximal cost-effectiveness. The authors used the two-injection technique, one on the right side and one on the left side of the celiac trunk. Patients were followed at monthly intervals during 24 weeks.

There were no major complications from the EUS-guided CPN in this series of patients. Five patients had a transient increase in abdominal pain and 9 patients had transient diarrhea lasting maximally one week. Almost 80% of patients noticed a reduction in their pain scores 2 weeks after CPN and the effect lasted for the entire study period of 24 weeks. Patients undergoing chemotherapeutic or radiotherapeutic adjuvant therapy had lower pain scores compared to patient without additional treatment during the follow-up period.

Only one comparative study between EUS-guided and another type of CPN (CT-guided) has been published [7]. This study, which included 22 patients, concerned patients with pain from benign chronic pancreatitis. The second major difference between this and other studies is the fact that patients were injected with triamcinolon instead of ethanol. Because of the benign character of their disease and the possibility of surgical procedures at a later stage of their disease, ethanol was considered to be contra-indicated because of the possibility of scarring and fibrosis. Eighteen patients could be evaluated in this study, 10 treated under EUS-guidance, 8 under CT-guidance. The overall results are less impressive than those reported in others studies. Seven out of eighteen patients had an improvement of their pain scores with an advantage for EUS-guided (50% improvement) over CT-guided CPN (25% improvement). The patients treated under EUS-guidance also had a longer lasting effect of their treatment. EUS-guided CPN was finally associated with less costs in this United States hospital (US $ 1,100 *vs* US $ 1,400). Also in this series, no serious side effects were noted.

Conclusions

EUS-guided celiac plexus neurolysis seems to be another excellent addition to the spectrum of interventional EUS. Its main indication is patients pancreatic cancer, where it may be performed quite early in the disease. The opportunity to diagnose, stage and treat the complications of pancreatic cancer during one endoscopic intervention clearly contributes to the attractivity of this procedure. The procedure can be easily and accurately performed by anyone with experience in EUS-guided fine needle aspiration biopsies, using the same instrument and same accessories. Because of the complexity of the palliative care of these patients, EUS-guided CPN should be integrated in the team approach to these patients. EUS-guided CPN should not be expected to replace morfinomimetics but to improve response to these medications.

References

1. Kappis M. Erfahrungen mit Lokalanaesthesie bei Bauchoperationen. *Vehr Dtsch Gesellsch Chir* 1914; 43: 87-9.
2. Gress F, Savides T, Cummings O, Sherman S, Lehman G, Zaidi S, *et al.* Radial scanning and linear array endosonography for staging pancreatic cancer: a prospective randomized comparison. *Gastrointest Endosc* 1997; 45: 138-42.
3. Wiersema MJ, Vilmann P, Giovannini M, Chang KJ, Wiersema LM. Endosonography-guided fine-needle apiration biopsy: Diagnostic accuracy and complication assessment. *Gastroenterology* 1997; 112: 1087-95.
4. Wiersema MJ, Wiersema LM. Endosonography-guided celiac plexus neurolysis. *Gastrointest Endosc* 1996; 44 (6): 656-62.
5. Lillemoe KD, Cameron JL, Kaufman HS, Yeo CJ, Pitt HA, Sauter PK. Chemical splanchnicectomy in patients with unresectable pancreatic cancer. A prospective randomized trial. *Ann Surg* 1993; 217: 447-57.
6. Gunaratnam NT, Sarma AV, Norton ID, Wiersema MJ. A prospective study of EUS-guided celiac plexus neurolysis for pancreatic cancer pain. *Gastrointest Endosc* 2001; 54: 316-24.
7. Gress F, Schmitt C, Sherman S, Ikenberry S, Lehman G. A prospective randomized comparison of endoscopic ultrasound- and computed tomography-guided celiac plexus block for managing chronic pancreatitis pain. *Am J Gastroenterol* 1999; 94: 900-5.

Cyst drainage procedures

Thierry Ponchon

Hépato-Gastroentérologie, Hôpital Édouard-Herriot, Lyon, France

Pseudocyst transmural drainage is one of the most demonstrative implications of therapeutic endoscopic ultrasound. But the series up to now are rather short and the need for EUS to perform transmural drainage of pseudocysts is still questioned, though EUS guidance carries theoretically many advantages.

Background

Traditionally, pancreatic pseudocysts have been treated initially with conservative management and surgery with internal drainage for those cases in which the pseudocyst does not resolve conservatively. On the other hand, drainage of pseudocyst has been conducted using endoscopy since 1975. However, the number of reported series of endoscopic drainage is still short due the limited number of indications and due to numerous prerequisites: before performing an endoscopic drainage of a pancreatic pseudocyst, the endoscopists should be aware of different considerations concerning the nature of the lesion, the relationship of the cyst with the pancreatic duct, the associated lesions... Six factors have to be clarified before opting for the endoscopic therapy:

1. **Misdiagnosis with a pancreatic cystic neoplasm should be avoided**. The diagnosis of cystic neoplasm, especially of mucinous cystadenoma or cystadenocarcinoma, or of intraductal papillary mucinous neoplasm must be first excluded, as surgical resection is usually indicated in these cases. Absence of alcohol abuse, absence of pancreatic calcifications must call attention and must question about the nature of the cystic lesion.

2. **An associated pseudoaneurysm should be sought**. Such pseudoaneuryms which have been described associated to pseudocysts in 10% of cases in certain series is the major

cause of severe bleeding following pseudocyst drainage. Mechanism of bleeding lies on the sudden decompression of the vascular lesion by the cyst drainage.

3. **A precise analysis of the pancreatic ducts must be conducted**: intraductal stone? Downstream ductal stricture? Communication between the ductal system and the pseudocyst? In these cases, an endoscopic drainage of the pancreatic duct or a transpapillary drainage of the cyst should be addressed prior transmural drainage, as persistence of intraductal stones or ductal stricture may result in cyst recurrence. The best plan is to insert a drain or a stent into the cyst through the papilla but at least, main pancreatic duct drainage can result in cyst resolution.

4. **The etiology of the cyst should be taken into consideration**: acute pancreatitis? Chronic pancreatitis? Concerning pseudocysts which complicate the course of chronic pancreatitis, endoscopic drainage is a valuable alternative to surgery while for pseudocysts due to acute pancreatitis, there is still a matter of controversy. These cysts are usually infected and contain debris and necrotic tissues, which are quasi impossible to drain or extract through the endoscopic tract. Endoscopic drainage of pseudocysts in case of acute pancreatitis related pseudocyst is less effective with more septic complications than in case of chronic pancreatitis related pseudocyst. Even if endoscopic drainage is performed, the persistence of necrotic tissues requires finally a large surgical drainage. Baron *et al.* [1] reported in 1996 a 50% morbidity rate and a high rate of repeated procedures in a series of 11 patients with necrotic pancreatic cyst and they recommended at least the use of nasocystic catheters to irrigate the cyst. Endoscopic drainage of cysts with large amounts of necrotic debris or prominent septae should not be attempted.

5. **The symptoms related to the cyst should be analyzed**. It is usually recommended to only treat pseudocysts with symptoms (pain) or complications (cholestasis due to bile duct compression, duodenal compression, portal or splenic vein compression, infection, pleural, mediastinal and peritoneal effusion). In the absence of symptoms or complications, the rule of 6 week waiting prior endoscopic drainage is debatted: some authors have demonstrated that spontaneous resolution of the cyst can occur very lately and do recommend to wait longer than 6 weeks. For other authors, a cyst diameter > 5 cm is a reliable indicator for drainage as it promotes non resolution of cyst and complications.

6. **Finally, another prerequisite is suitable anatomy**. The relationship of the cyst with the enteral wall is a major factor to be evaluated. Some pseudocysts have a close and direct apposition to the enteral wall and cause bulging of the stomach or duodenum; but some cysts are developped at a distance from the wall and of course are more difficult or impossible to drain transmurally. Classically, the distance between the cyst and the gut wall should not exceed 10 mm. The shortest distance between the cyst and the wall should be determined. Some vessels, especially in case of associated portal hypertension, can be interposed between the digestive wall and the cyst inducing a risk of bleeding. Relation to the neighboring structures has thus to be assessed: gastric varices and summucosal vessels using colour Doppler examination, digestive structures, peritoneum (perforation).

For all these reasons, endoscopic cyst drainage should not be attempted without a complete evaluation of the cyst and the surrounding tissues by US, EUS with colour doppler examination, CT-scan, MRCP and if necessary retrograde wirsungography.

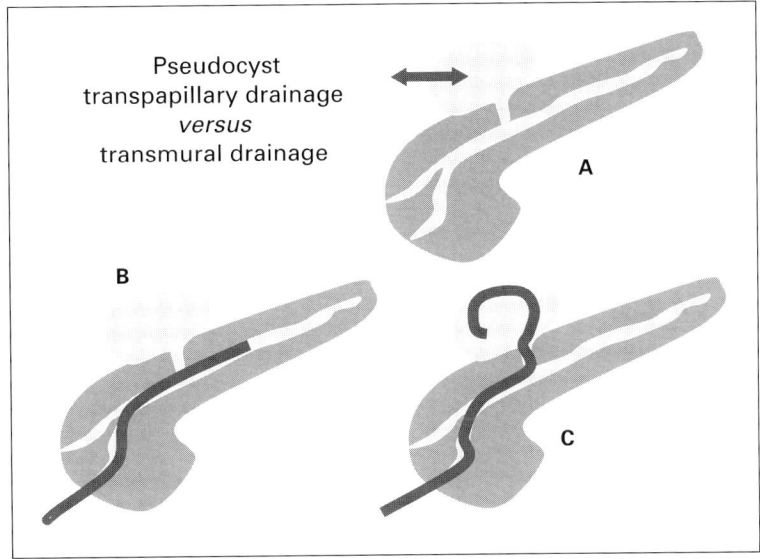

Figure 1. Diagram of the different methods of endoscopic pseudocyst drainage. A: Transmural drainage of the cyst. B: Transpapillary drainage of the main pancreatic duct. C: Transpapillary drainage of the cyst.

Table I. Endoscopic therapy of pancreatic pseudocysts: series without EUS guidance.

	Type of drainage	Number of patients	Immediate success (%)	Complications (%)	Follow-up duration	Late success (%)
Cremer, 1989 [2]	CE	33	98	13	31 months	82
Sahel, 1991 [3]	CE	52		15		72
Monkemuller, 1998 [4]	CE	94	94	12		
Kozarek, 1991 [5]	TP	18	89	22	16 months	78
Catalano, 1995 [6]	TP	21	81	4	37 months	76
Barthet, 1995 [7]	TP	30	87	10	15 months	
Dohmoto, 1992 [8]	TP + CE	17	100	6		84
Binmoeller, 1995 [9]	TP + CE	24	86	10	22 months	87
Smits, 1995 [10]	TP + CE	37	92	16	32 months	65
Howell, 1998 [11]	TP + CE	64	94	24	10 months	67
Vitale, 1999 [12]	TP + CE	29			13 months	83
Beckingham, 1999 [13]	TP + CE	34	71	18	46 months	62

KE: cystenterostomy, TP: transpapillary drainage.

More than 400 cases of endoscopically managed pseudocysts have been reported. The results of the different series [2-13] are presented in *Table I*. Endoscopic therapy is associated with a high technical success rate, acceptable low rate of complications, and a recurrence rate of 20-30%. In *Table I*, the type of drainage, transmural or transpapillary has been specified: it appears that the success rate and the morbidity rate are not different between both methods. The transpapillary drainage carries less risks of bleeding and perforation but has a higher rate of infection.

Although several techniques of transmural drainage have been described, the principle is unique consisting to create a communication between the cyst and the digestive lumen and usually to let in place a double pigtail stent to maintain patency of the cystenterostomy. The incidence of complications may have been higher in the earlier series because of the technique of extending the fistula by using a papillotome. This technique has been abandonned and replaced by stent insertion. Monkemuller *et al.* [4] presented in 1998 a large retrospective series of 94 cases of transmural drainage. They used both needle-knife entry technique (43 patients) and Seldinger technique without electrocautery (51 patients). Success rate was almost identical for both techniques but Seldinger technique carries less complications (4.6%) than the needle-knife method (15.7%).

Finally, it is very difficult from the litterature to compare the results between cystgastrostomy and cystduodenostomy: we get enough data only from 2 series [2, 10]). Morbidity rate, especially infection rate, is higher (33%) with cystgastrostomy than with cystduodenostomy and long-term success rate is lower (52% *versus* 89%). Different reasons for this discrepancy are suggested: the cysts apposed to the gastric wall are usually large, with a declive component, leading to stasis, especially stasis of food debris from the stomach. For some authors, the role of endoscopic cystogastrostomy is still discussed.

The role of EUS

The role of EUS during endoscopic transmural drainage of pseudocyst is obvious owing to the anatomical difficulties pointed out above. EUS is helpful to determine:
– the nature and the content of the cyst,
– the distance between the digestive wall and the cyst,
– the presence of intervening vessels and of neighboring structures which have to be avoided,
– and finally the optimal and safe site for drainage, *i.e.* the shortest route between the digestive wall and the cyst, without intervening vessels.

The role of EUS has enlarged in accordance with the advances in EUS technology. Three steps can be distinguished in the history of EUS guided therapy of pancreatic pesudocysts.

Initial method [14]

EUS has been used initially to overcome the blind nature of the traditional endoscopic procedure. EUS is conducted prior inserting a large operating channel gastroscope or

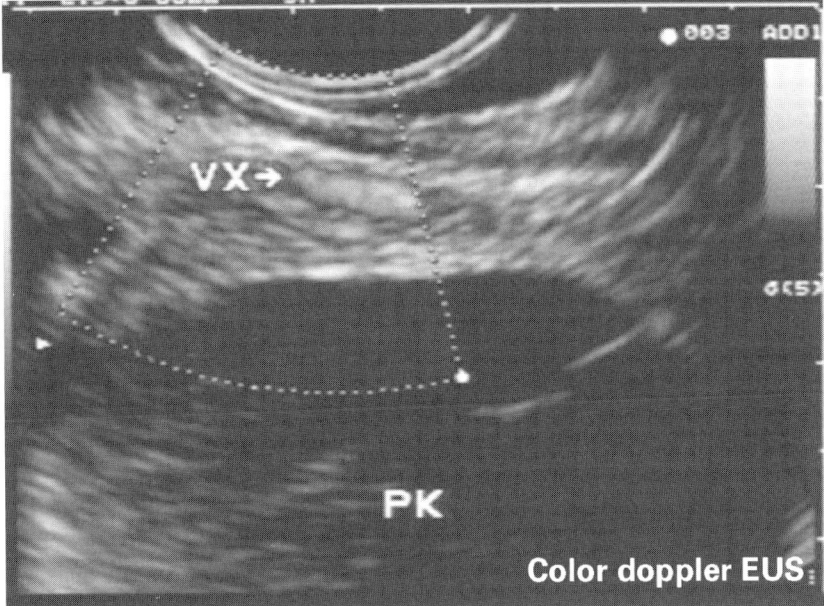

Figure 2. EUS Color doppler image of pseudocyst (PK). Color doppler clearly demonstrates a vessel interposed between the pseudocyst and the digestive wall. This site is thus contraindicated for puncture (M. Giovannini).

duodenoscope. The optimal site of the drainage is selected by EUS and marked, for example, by biopsy forceps bite or dye injection. This is a semiblind method, as the puncture and the drainage are not totally controlled by EUS. But at least EUS allows puncturing pseudocyst more safely even without luminal bulging. A report of Gerolami *et al.* [15] on 4 patients illustrates that in some cases, EUS may contraindicate endoscopic attempts, while in others it may guide puncture. Fockens *et al.* [16] performed EUS in 32 patients referred for pseudocyst drainage and observed that EUS leads to a change of therapy in 37.5% of patients. As indicated above, surgical decompression is still considered the treatment of choice for infected pseudocyst, but Fuchs *et al.* [17] have reported recently three cases of patients with infected pseudocyst treated succesfully by EUS guided method.

Intermediate method [18]

Once curved array transducer US endoscopes with operating channel were commercially available, the pseudocyst could be punctured directly under EUS guidance using a diathermic needle. The method consists then to insert a guide-wire through the needle into the cyst. The EUS scope is withdrawn and a large channel duodenoscope is introduced on the guide-wire to perform a large diameter stent insertion through the wall. This technique is time-consuming, especially if the wire slips out during the exchange of intruments.

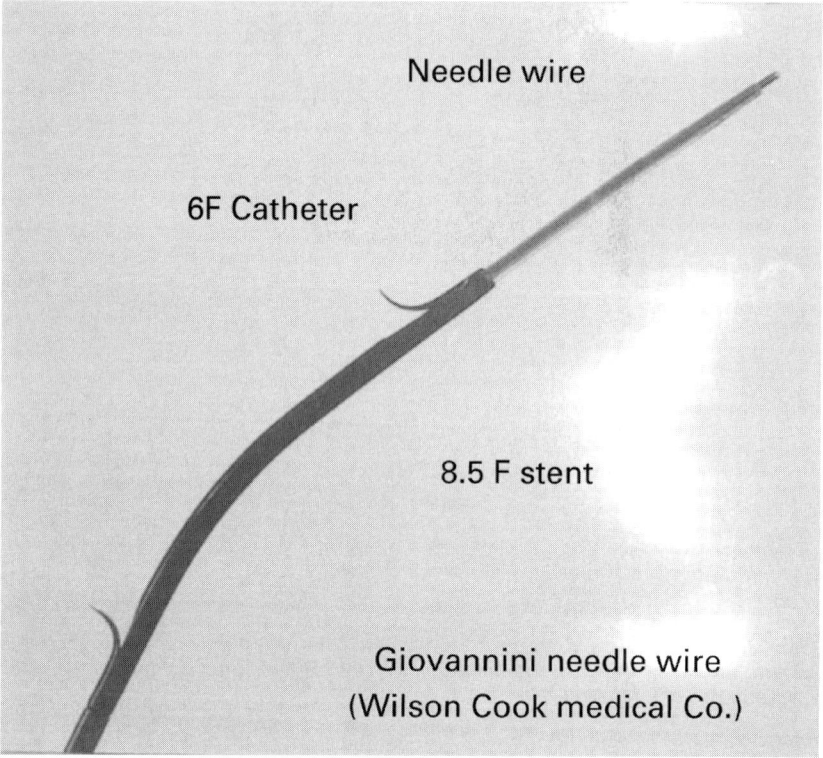

Figure 3. Dedicated device for one-step EUS-guided drainage of pseudocyst.

Final method

The cyst drainage is conducted exclusively by EUS, avoiding exchange of endoscopes. This step is based on the use of a dedicated large channel EUS scope and of a dedicated stent delivery system. The operating channel diameter is usually 3.2 mm. Vilmann *et al.* [19] reported in 1998 the first case of one-step EUS-guided transmural drainage of a pseudocyst. They used EUS all along the procedure and therefore they employed a large channel prototype EUS scope and a special delivery system, which permitted in the same time to perform the cystenterostomy and to insert a 8.5 French double pigtail stent. The delivery system ready to be introduced in the operating channel of the scope had a metal diathermy tip, a plastic catheter and the stent mounted on the plastic catheter. The system was advanced by means of a handle piston close to the wall. Then diathermy needle activated by cutting current penetrated into the cystic cavity, followed by the plastic catheter and the stent. The double pigtail stent was then released by withdrawal of the plastic catheter. The method was successful in this case resulting in a 6 cm diameter cyst collapse. The authors explained that the large diameter and the stiffness of the scope were not disadvantageous, as they helped to stabilize the scope during the puncture and the stent introduction.

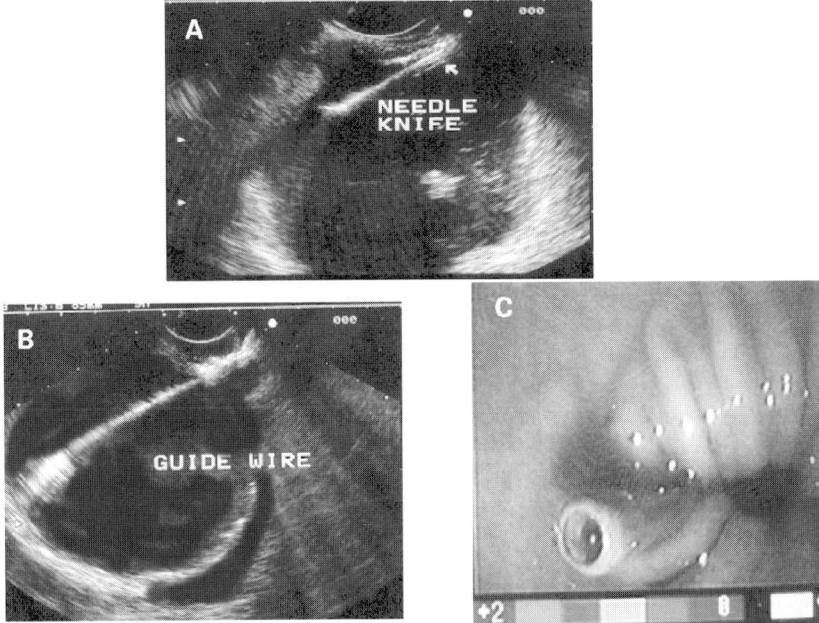

Figure 4. Different steps during the endoscopic EUS guided drainage of a pseudocyst (M. Giovannini). A: EUS control: a pseudocyst is apposed to the gastric wall and the needle-wire has been inserted in the cyst under EUS guidance. B: EUS control of drainage: a guide-wire has been introduced through the needle into the cyst. C: Endoscopic control: a 8.5F stent has been inserted between the gastric lumen and the pseudocyst.

Then Giovannini et al. [20] described their experience with cystgastrostomy guided exclusively using EUS in 6 patients. Two patients had a chronic pancreatitis and for 4 patients, the cyst was a complication of an acute pancreatitis. None of the cysts was bulging into the gastric lumen. Giovannini et al. did not use a special device for stent delivery. They first opened the wall with a needle-knife. Once the needle-knife was into the cyst, the metal wire of the knife was withdrawn leaving a teflon catheter in place. A guide-wire was then introduced into the cyst through the teflon catheter and on the guide-wire a 8 French stent or a 7 French nasocystic drain was inserted. Catheter or stent insertion was successful in 5 cases. In one case, only a puncture was performed. Finally, only one recurrence due a stent obstruction was observed and treated by stent exchange.

Seifert et al [21] also reported recently transmural drainage of cystic abdominal lesions using a one-step EUS-guided method. They developed a dedicated needle-stent device. The needle was 1 mm large and no electrocautery was used to facilitate the insertion of a 7 F stent which was pushed on the needle. Six patients were treated (2 with chronic pancreatitis, 3 with acute pancreatitis and one with an abcess) and 5 had satisfactory results. Baron et al. [22] recently described the first case of EUS-guided transesophageal pancreatic pseudocyst drainage. This case illustrated the role of EUS to select the more suitable and safer site for drainage.

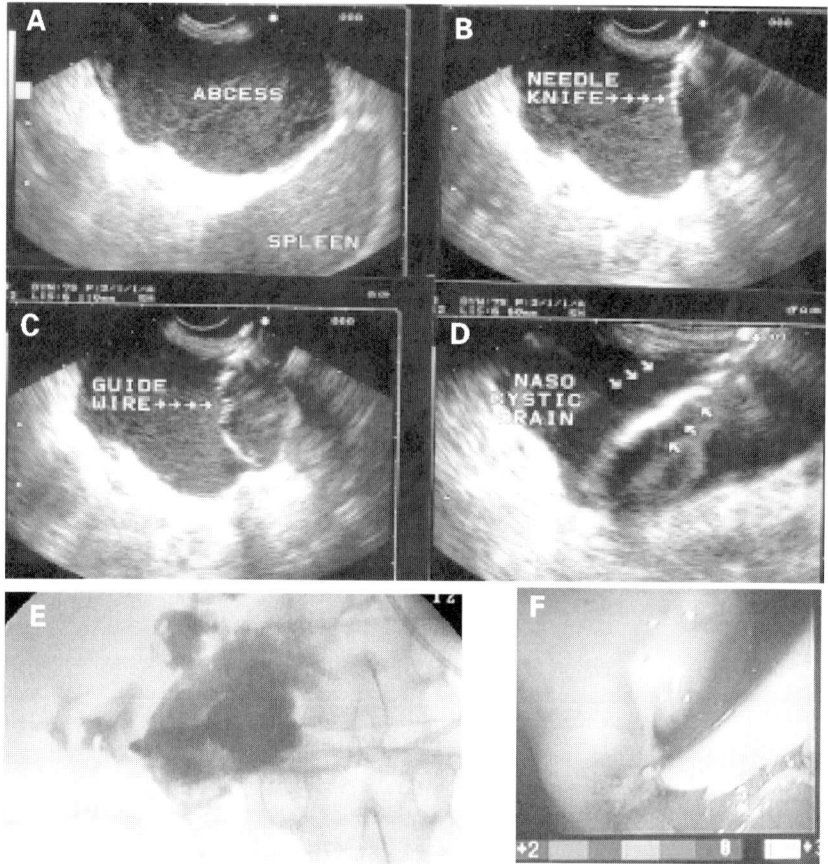

Figure 5. Different steps during the EUS guided drainage of a pancreatic abscess (M. Giovannini). A: Heterogeneous content of the cyst. B: Introduction of the needle. C: Introduction of the guide-wire through the needle. D: Introduction of the nasocystic catheter on the guide-wire. The distal shape of the catheter is easily recognizable. E: Fluoroscopic view of the drain in place in the pancreatic abscess. F: Endoscopic view of the drain.

The more recent publication is from Giovannini *et al.* [23]: they treated 35 patients, 15 with chronic pancreatitis related pseudocyst and 20 with post-operative acute pancreatitis related abscesses. They employed the method described above, plus a dilation of the tract using a 8 mm balloon. For pseudocyst, a 8.5 F stent was inserted, while for abscess, a 7 F nasocystic catheter was let in place 8-10 days for irrigation. Placement of stents or catheters was achieved in 18/20 abscesses and 10/10 pseudocysts. Over a mean follow-up of 27 months, one cyst and 2 abscesses recurred. Overall success rate was thus 88.5%.

At this moment, disadvantage of the one-step EUS guided method is the limited size of the stent. Improved endoscope and accessories that allow placement of 10 F double pigtail stent will likely to be developed.

Conclusion

If EUS is mandatory for planning therapy of pancreatic pseudocysts, the role of EUS during drainage is still controversed. No controlled studies have been conducted to demonstrate that EUS reduces the morbidity rate of the procedure, but the more recent series are very encouraging due to the technological progresses accomplished on the scopes and leads to recommend systematic EUS guidance of pseudocyst transmural drainage.

References

1. Baron TH, Thaggard WG, Morgan DE, Stanley RJ. Endoscopic therapy for organized pancreatic necrosis. *Gastroenterology* 1996; 111: 755-64.
2. Cremer M, Deviere J, Engelhom L. Endoscopic management of cysts and pseudocysts in chronic pancreatitis. Long-term follow-up after 7 years of experience. *Gastrointest Endosc* 1989; 35: 1-9.
3. Sahel J. Endoscopic drainage of pancreatic cysts. *Endoscopy* 1991; 23: 181-4.
4. Monkemuller KE, Baron TH, Morgan DE. Transmural drainage of pancreatic fluid collections without electrocautery using the Seldinger technique. *Gastrointest Endosc* 1998; 48: 195-200.
5. Kozarek RA, Ball TJ, Patterson DJ, Freeny PC, Ryan JA, Traverso LW. Endoscopic transpapillary therapy for disrupted pancreatic duct and peripancreatic fluid collections. *Gastroenterology* 1991; 100: 1362-70.
6. Catalano MF, Geenen JE, Schmalz MJ, Johnson GK, Dean RS, Hogan WJ. Treatment of pancreatic pseudocysts with ductal communication by transpapillary pancreatic duct endoprosthesis. *Gastrointest Endosc* 1995; 42: 214-8.
7. Barthet M, Sahel J, Bodiou-Bertei C, Bernard JP. Endoscopic transpapillary drainage of pancreatic pseudocysts. *Gastrointest Endosc* 1995; 42: 208-13.
8. Dohmoto M, Rupp KD. Endoscopic drainage of pancreatic pseudocysts. *Surg Endosc* 1992; 6: 118-24.
9. Binmoeller KF, Seifert H, Walter A, Soehendra N. Transpapillary and transmural drainage of pancreatic pseudocysts. *Gastrointest Endosc* 1995; 42: 219-24.
10. Smits ME, Rauws EAJ, Tytgat GNJ, Huibregste K. The efficacy of endoscopic treatment of pancreatic pseudocysts. *Gastrointest Endosc* 1995; 42: 202-7.
11. Howell DA, Elton E, Parsons WG. Endoscopic management of pseudocysts of pancreas. *Gastrointest Endosc Clin North Am* 1998; 8: 143-62.
12. Vitale GC, Lawhon JC, Larson GM, Harrell DJ, Reed DN Jr, MacLeod S. Endoscopic drainage of the pancreatic pseudocyst. *Surgery* 1999; 126: 616-21.
13. Beckingham IJ, Krige JE, Bornman PC, Terblanche J. Endoscopic management of pancreatic pseudocysts. *Br J Surg* 1997; 84: 1638-45.
14. Grimm H, Binmoeller KF, Soehendra N. Endosonography-guided drainage of a pancreatic pseudocyst. *Gastrointest Endosc* 1992; 38: 170-1.
15. Gerolami R, Giovannini M, Laugier R. Endoscopic drainage of pancreatic pseudocysts guided by endosonography. *Endoscopy* 1997; 29: 106-8.
16. Fockens P, Johnson TG, Van Dullemen HM, Huibregste K, Tytgat GN. Endosonographic imaging of pancreatic pseudocysts before endoscopic transmural drainage. *Gastrointest Endosc* 1997; 46: 412-6.
17. Fuchs M, Reimann FM, Gaebel C, Ludwig D, Stagne EF. Treatment of infected pancreactic pseudocysts by endoscopic ultrasonography-guided cystogastrostomy. *Endoscopy* 2000; 32: 654-7.
18. Wiersema MJ. Endosonography-guided cystoduodenostomy with a therapeutic ultrasound endoscope. *Gastrointest Endosc* 1996; 44: 614-7.

19. Vilmann P, Hancke S, Pless T, Schell-Hincke JD, Henriksen FW. One-step endosonography-guided drainage of a pancreatic pseudocyst: a new technique of stent delivery through the echo endoscope. *Endoscopy* 1998; 30: 730-3.
20. Giovannini M, Bernardini D, Seitz JF. Cystogastrostomy entirely performed under endosonography guidance for panacreatic pseudocyst: results in 6 patients. *Gastrointest Endosc* 1998; 48: 200-3.
21. Seifert H, Dietrich C, Schmitt T, Caspary W, Wehrmann T. Endoscopic utrasound-guided one-step transmural drainage of cystic abdominal lesions with a large-channel echo endoscope. *Endoscopy* 2000; 32: 255-9.
22. Baron Th, Wiersema MJ. EUS-guided transesophageal pancreatic pseudocyst drainage. *Gastrointest Endosc* 2000; 52: 545-9.
23. Giovannini M, Pesenti C, Rolland AL, Moutardier V, Delpero JR. Endoscopic ultrasound-guided drainage of pancreatic pseudocysts or pancreatic abscesses using a therapeutic echo endoscope. *Endoscopy* 2001; 33: 473-7.

IV

Endoscopic Procedures for Palliation

Treatment of malignant colonic stenosis with self-expandable metallic stents

Richard A. Kozarek

Section of Gastroenterology, Virginia Mason Medical Center, Seattle, WA, USA

Historically, the nonsurgical treatment of malignant gastrointestinal stenoses was limited to accessible areas, namely, the esophagus and anorectum [1]. The former included bougienage and rigid prosthesis insertion while the latter, periodic dilation and snare debulking of neoplasm in high-surgical-risk patients. Later, large channel duodenoscopes allowed insertion of plastic prostheses to bypass obstructing pancreaticobiliary neoplasms in a subset of patients with unresectable disease. It was later still that the development and application of ablative modalities endoscopically, particularly Nd-YAG laser, but also multipolar cautery, caustic injection, and photodynamic therapy, allowed treatment of more central stenoses. Concomitant with these developments were the introduction and widespread application of through-the-scope (TTS) dilating balloons. Thus, a variety of benign and malignant stenoses which were previously inaccessible became theoretically amenable to endotherapy, either with dilation alone or dilation followed by application of an ablative modality. Conventional stents could not be inserted in most malignant central stenoses (small bowel, colon) because of the length of the delivery systems and the acute angulation of many of the stenoses.

It was the development of expandable prostheses, however, that allowed, at least in theory, a technique to establish more permanent luminal patency without recourse to surgery [2]. Used initially in the biliary tree and later in the esophagus, these prostheses have variably supplanted more conventional stents, especially in the esophagus [3]. Purported advantages, contingent upon stent design, include ability to conform to angulated anatomy, obviating aggressive dilation during the placement phase, and tissue ingrowth to preclude migration [4-12].

While there are now ample data to show that expandable stents maintain patency in the biliary tree longer than conventional prostheses [13-15], and that expandable stents may be easier and safer to insert into the esophagus when compared to conventional ones, no controlled studies have demonstrated that their insertion confers survival advantage to these unfortunate patients [16]. Moreover, there are now numerous studies demonstrating long-term complications related to expandable stent therapy. The latter include, but are not limited to: bleeding; migration; erosion; tumor ingrowth or overgrowth; elicitation of mucosal hyperplasia or granulation tissue; food impaction; stent impaction upon the contralateral wall; and prosthesis fracture [10, 13, 17-23].

Expandable stents for colonic stenosis

It is upon this background that expandable stent therapy for central GI stenoses must build. To date, most of the studies published have borrowed prostheses originally designed for the biliary tree or the esophagus and most lack design or insertion characteristics of true central stents. Prostheses that have been used include the enteral Wallstent® (Microvasive, Inc., Natick, MA) 18-20 mm in diameter, 6-9 cm in length, and the only expandable prosthesis designed to be placed through a large channel endoscope; CoRectCoil® (IntraTherapeutics, Eden-Prairie, MN); Z® stent (Wilson-Cook, Inc., Winston-Salem, NC); the Ultraflex® (Microvasive, Inc., Natick, MA); Memotherm (Bard, Inc., Billerica, MA); and the Choostent (MI Tech, Seoul, Korea) *(Table 1)*. All of the latter have been designed primarily for the esophagus and/or biliary tree. As such, the esophagus delivery systems are often too short or rigid to allow deployment to treat malignant obstructions at the splenic flexure or beyond. Moreover, the diameter of the biliary stents (6 to 10 mm) make the biliary forms of these prostheses unsatisfactory to maintain colonic integrity. Finally, the physical characteristics of the above-mentioned prostheses make all of them suboptimal for central stenoses. Thus, Z® stents are relatively rigid and fail to conform to acutely angulated stenoses. Wallstents® and Ultraflex® stents allow tumor ingrowth and the exposed wires of the Wallstent® are often associated with not only elicitation of granulation tissue proximally and distally, but also local perforation. The EsophaCoil® (CoRectCoil®), in turn, may entrap mucosal folds between loops of the prosthesis and the extremely high radial force may be associated with acute or subsequent perforation of a tight malignant stenosis [1].

Table I. Self-expandable metallic stents (SEMS) marketed/utilized for colonic stenoses

SEMS	Available lengths (cm)	Stent diameters (mm)	Length delivery catheter (cm)	Delivery catheter size (F)	Material
Enteral Wallstent®	6, 9	18, 20, 22	135, 255	10	Elgiloy
CoRectCoil®	7.5, 10	18, 20	80	32	Nitinol
Z®	4, 6, 8, 10, 12	25	40	31	Stainless steel
Choostent®	8, 11, 14, 17	22	75, 120	12	Nitinol
Memotherm®	6, 8, 10	25, 30	120	14.5	Nitinol

It should also be emphasized that, in contrast to studies that have been done in the esophagus [7, 8], and at least with plastic prostheses in the biliary tree [24, 25], there are no series randomizing patients with colonic obstruction with traditional therapy (*i.e.* surgical bypass or resection). Nor, unlike previous studies with malignant esophageal obstruction, are there studies randomizing stent therapy compared with ablative modalities such as laser or photodynamic therapy (PDT). As such, all of the papers published at this time utilizing expandable stents for malignant central stenoses, including our own, are "home movies", uncontrolled observations in an unfortunate and often high-surgical-risk patient population.

Results in colon obstruction

Comparable to self-expandable metallic stents (SEMS) application for gastric outlet obstruction, there have been no randomized studies that have compared palliative stent placement with surgical resection or diversion in patients with colonic obstruction in the setting of metastatic disease. Nor are there studies that have randomized stent placement preoperatively to two stage diversion and resection in resectable patients with acute, malignant obstruction. Nor has prosthesis insertion been compared to urgent lumen recanalization using laser photoablation, pneumatic dilation alone, BICAP coagulation, or cryotherapy [26-28].

Instead, there have been small, single institution series, often using a variety of prostheses not designed for colonic placement *(Table II)*. In one, Baron *et al.* published some sobering results [29]. They placed various types of prostheses in 25 patients (15 palliative, 10 in an attempt to decompress an acutely obstructed colon preoperatively). There was a 94% placement success and 85% of the prostheses were "effective". However, at a mean follow-up of 17 weeks (2 to 64), there was a 30% rate of stent migration, occlusion, or perforation. A larger series by Camuñez *et al.* demonstrated procedural efficacy in 70 of 80 patients with malignant bowel obstruction and symptomatic resolution in 67 (96%) [30]. There were 2 procedural perforations and in the 35 patients in whom SEMS were used for palliation, the patency rate at 3 and 6 months was 91%. Survival rate for this palliative group was 55% at 3, 44% at 6, and 25% at 9 months, respectively. In contrast, in a multicenter trial reported by DeGregorio *et al.*, 23 of 24 (96%) of patients resolved acute colonic obstruction after SEMS placement, although 42% of patients ultimately developed complications [31]. Additional series using expandable prostheses in the colon have been reported by Binkert *et al.* [32], Feretis *et al.* [33], Spinelli and Mancini [34], Repecici *et al.* [35], Cole *et al.* [36], Herrero *et al.* [37], Miyayama *et al.* [38], Liberman *et al.* [39], Law *et al.* [40], Tamin *et al.* [41], and our group [42].

In addition to the above, Tack *et al.* reported 10 patients with advanced obstructing rectosigmoid carcinoma initially treated with Nd-YAG laser followed by attempted Ultraflex® stent insertion [43]. Following a mean of 2 ± 0.4 laser sessions, minimal luminal diameter approximated 9 ± 1 mm. Stents were successfully placed in 9 patients with resultant luminal diameter of 14 ± 1.2 mm ($p < 0.005$). There was a single colon perforation during one of the stent insertion attempts and 3 prostheses migrated at a mean 38 ± 10 days. Patient survival approximated 204 ± 43 days and a single patient developed subsequent tumor ingrowth. Comparable data have been published by Rey *et al.* using laser in conjunction with Wallstent® placement [44].

Finally, in one of the largest series to date, Mainar *et al.* placed 72 stents in 71 patients with malignant colon obstruction [45]. There was a 90% technical success rate, a 13%

Table II. Selected series using self-expandable metallic stents (SEMS) for malignant colorectal obstruction

	Stent type	#Pts	Success (%)	Palliation/ Prep	Effectiveness (%)	Complications (%)
Baron et al. [29]	Variable	25	94	17/10*	85	30
Binkert et al. [32]	Ultraflex	13	92	3/10	83	23
Spinelli et al. [34]	Z	37	97	28/9	78	22
Mainar et al. [45]	Wallstent/ Memotherm	71	90	0/71	93	14
DeGregorio et al. [31]	Variable	24	96	9/15	96	42
Camuñez et al. [30]	Wallstent	80	88	35/33**	91	10

* Intent to treat analysis
** Patients with successful/uncomplicated SEMS insertion

minor complication rate and a single perforation requiring urgent operation. All patients underwent surgery at a mean of 8.6 days (6-16 days) post SEMS. These and additional data are synopsized in several recent or upcoming review articles [46-50].

Conclusions

It is the author's opinion that colonic stenting is still in its infancy and, accordingly, use in benign disease should be discouraged. Despite refinements in both prostheses and delivery systems, none are ideal for central stenoses and it is unlikely that one technology will be adaptable to all anatomic or pathologic situations. The goal for the future, then, is one of refining prostheses and their insertion devices in an attempt to minimize perforations, migrations, and granulation tissue, tumor overgrowth or ingrowth. Possibilities include tighter weave stents without exposed proximal and distal wires, prostheses fabricated of material that may actually be incorporated into as opposed to imbedding in tissue, mucosal paving techniques, or stents that are used as delivery devices of chemotherapeutic drugs. Additional goals are modeled after studies already conducted with esophageal neoplasm [51]. They include better definition of which stent should be used and in which situation as well as the relative role of prostheses when compared to conventional surgery, interventional radiology, or current and future transendoscopic ablative techniques.

References

1. Kozarek RA. Gastrointestinal stenting. In: Yamada T, Alpers DH, Owyang C, Powell DW, Laine L, eds. *Textbook of Gastroenterology* (volume II) (3rd ed.), Philadelphia: JB Lippincott Co., 1999: 2811-24.
2. Kozarek RA. Expandable endoprostheses for gastrointestinal stenoses. *Gastrointest Endosc Clin North Am* 1994; 4: 279-95.
3. Kozarek RA. Use of expandable stents for esophageal and biliary stenoses. *Gastroenterologist* 1994; 2: 264-72.

4. Winkelbauer FW, Schöfl R, Niederle B, et al. Palliative treatment of obstructing cancer with nitinol stents: value, safety, and long-term results. *Am J Radiol* 1996; 166: 79-84.
5. Shim CS, Yee YH, Cho YD, et al. Preliminary results of a new covered biliary metal stent for malignant biliary obstruction. *Endoscopy* 1998; 30: 345-50.
6. Goldin E, Bayar M, Safra T, et al. A new self-expandable and removable metal stent for biliary obstruction – a preliminary report. *Endoscopy* 1993; 25: 597-9.
7. Siersma PP, Hop WCJ, Dees J, et al. Coated self-expanding metal stents versus latex prostheses for esophagogastric cancer with special reference to prior radiation and chemotherapy. A controlled prospective study. *Gastrointest Endosc* 1998; 47: 113-20.
8. Knyrim K, Wagner HJ, Bethge N, et al. A controlled trial of expansile metal stents for palliation of esophageal obstruction due to inoperable cancer. *N Engl J Med* 1993; 329: 1302-7.
9. Kozarek RA, Raltz S, Brugge WR, et al. Prospective multicenter trial of esophageal Z-stent placement for malignant dysphagia and tracheoesophageal fistula. *Gastrointest Endosc* 1996; 44: 562-7.
10. Nelson DB, Axelrad AM, Fleischer DE, et al. Silicone covered Wallstent prototypes for palliation of malignant esophageal obstruction and digestive-respiratory fistulas. *Gastrointest Endosc* 1997; 45: 31-7.
11. Fan Z, Dai N, Chen L. Expandable thermal-shaped memory metal esophageal stent: experiences with a new nitinol stent in 129 patients. *Gastrointest Endosc* 1997; 46: 352-6.
12. May A, Hahn E, Ell C. Self-expanding metal stents for palliation of malignant obstruction in the upper gastrointestinal tract. Comparative assessment of three stent types implemented in 96 implantation. *J Clin Gastroenterol* 1996; 22: 201-6.
13. Carr-Locke DL, Connors PJ, Cotton PB, et al. Randomized prospective trial of plastic versus Wallstents for malignant biliary stricture. *Gastrointest Endosc* 1993; 39: 310 (abstract).
14. Davids PHP, Groen AK, Rauns EAJ, et al. A new self-expandable metal stent for biliary obstruction. *Gastrointest Endosc* 1992; 40: 1488-92.
15. Wagner HJ, Knyrim K, Vakil N, Klose KJ. Plastic endoprostheses versus metal stents in the palliative treatment of malignant hilar biliary obstruction. A prospective and randomized trial. *Endoscopy* 1993; 25: 213-8.
16. Kozarek RA, Ball TJ, Brandabur JJ, et al. Expandable versus conventional esophageal prostheses: easier insertion may not preclude subsequent stent-related problems. *Gastrointest Endosc* 1996; 43: 204-8.
17. Kozarek RA, Raltz S, Marcon N, et al. Use of the 25 mm flanged esophageal Z-stent for malignant dysphagia: a prospective multicenter trial. *Gastrointest Endosc* 1997; 46: 156-60.
18. Wengrower D, Fiorini A, Valero J, et al. EsophaCoil: long-term results in 81 patients. *Gastrointest Endosc* 1998; 48: 376-82.
19. Raijman I, Siddique I, Ajani J, Lynch P. Palliation of malignant dysphagia and fistulae with coated expandable metal stents: experience with 101 patients. *Gastrointest Endosc* 1998; 48: 172-9.
20. Schmassmann A, Meyenberger C, Knuchel J, et al. Self-expanding metal stents in malignant esophageal obstruction: a comparison between two stent types. *Am J Gastroenterol* 1997; 92: 400-6.
21. Nevitt AW, Kozarek RA, Conti N, et al. Complications encountered with use of expandable esophageal prostheses. *App Radiol* 1999.
22. Kozarek RA, Ball TJ, Patterson DJ. Metallic self-expanding stent application in the upper gastrointestinal tract: caveats and concerns. *Gastrointest Endosc* 1992; 38: 1-6.
23. Bethge N, Sommer A, Gross U, et al. Human tissue responses to metal stents implanted in vivo for the palliation of malignant stenoses. *Gastrointest Endosc* 1996; 43: 596-602.
24. Naggar E, Krag E, Matzen P. Endoscopically inserted biliary endoprostheses in malignant obstructive jaundice: a survey of the literature. *Liver* 1990; 10: 320-4.
25. Smith AC, Dowsett JF, Russell RCG. Randomized trial of endoscopic stenting versus surgical bypass in malignant low bile duct obstruction. *Lancet* 1994; 344: 1655-60.

26. Arrigoni A, Pannazio M, Spandre M, Rossini FP. Emergency endoscopy: recanalization of intestinal obstruction caused by colorectal cancer. *Gastrointest Endosc* 1994; 40: 576-88.
27. Heborer G, Denecke H, Demmel N, Wirshing R. Local procedures in the management of rectal cancer. *World J Surg* 1987; 11: 499-503.
28. Sander R. Photodynamic therapy in gastroenterology. *Gastroenterologist* 1994; 2: 180-3.
29. Baron TH, Dean PA, Yates MR 3rd, *et al*. Expandable metal stents for the treatment of colonic obstruction: technique and outcomes. *Gastrointest Endosc* 1998; 47: 277-85.
30. Camuñez F, Echenagusia A, Simó G, *et al*. Malignant colorectal obstruction treated by means of self-expanding metallic stents: effectiveness before surgery and in palliation. *Radiology* 2000; 216: 492-7.
31. DeGregorio MA, Mainar A, Tejero E, *et al*. Acute colorectal obstruction: stent placement for palliative treatment – results of a multicenter study. *Radiology* 1998; 209: 117-20.
32. Binkert CA, Ledermann H, Jost R, *et al*. Acute colonic obstruction: clinical aspects and cost-effectiveness of preoperative and palliative treatment with self-expanding metallic stents – a preliminary report. *Radiology* 1998; 206: 199-204.
33. Feretis C, Benakis P, Dimopoulos C, *et al*. Palliation of large bowel obstruction due to recurrent rectosigmoid tumor using self-expandable endoprostheses. *Endoscopy* 1996; 28: 319-22.
34. Spinelli P, Mancini A. Use of self-expanding metal stents for the palliation of rectosigmoid cancer. *Gastrointest Endosc* 2001; 53: 203-6.
35. Repici A, Reggio D, De Angelis C, *et al*. Covered metal stents for management of inoperable malignant colorectal stricture. *Gastrointest Endosc* 2000; 52: 735-40.
36. Cole SJ, Boorman P, Osman H, *et al*. Endoluminal stenting for relief of colorectal obstruction is safe and effective. *Colorectal Dis* 2000; 2: 282-7.
37. Herrero G, Diaz P, Pabon P, Fernandez LR. Placement of a colonic stent by percutaneous colostomy in a case of malignant stenosis. *Cardiovasc Intervent Radiol* 2001; 24: 67-9.
38. Miyayama S, Matsui O, Kitane K, *et al*. Malignant colonic obstruction due to extensive tumor: palliative treatment with a self-expanding nitinol stent. *Am J Roentgenol* 2000; 175: 1631-7.
39. Liberman H, Adams DR, Blatchford GJ, *et al*. Clinical use of the self-expanding metallic stent in the management of colorectal cancer. *Am J Surg* 2000; 180: 407-12.
40. Law WL, Chu KW, Ho JW, *et al*. Self-expanding metallic stent in the treatment of colonic obstruction caused by advanced malignancies. *Dis Colon Rectum* 2000; 43: 1522-7.
41. Tamin WZ, Ghellai A, Coanihan TC, *et al*. Experience with endoluminal colonic Wallstents for the management of large bowel obstruction for benign and malignant disease. *Arch Surg* 2000; 135: 434-8.
42. Kozarek RA, Brandabur JJ, Raltz SL. Expandable stents: unusual locations. *Am J Gastroenterol* 1997; 92: 812-5.
43. Tack J, Gevers AM, Rutgeerts P. Self-expandable metallic stents in the palliation of rectosigmoidal carcinoma: a follow-up study. *Gastrointest Endosc* 1998; 48: 267-71.
44. Rey SF, Romancyk T, Goeff M. Metal stents for palliation of rectal carcinoma: a preliminary report on 12 patients. *Endoscopy* 1995; 27: 501-4.
45. Mainar A, Ariza MA, Tejero E, *et al*. Acute colorectal obstruction: treatment with self-expandable metallic stents before scheduled surgery - results of a multicenter study. *Radiology* 1999; 210: 65-9.
46. Zollikofer CL, Jost R, Schoch E, Decurtins M. Gastrointestinal stenting (Review article). *Eur Radiol* 2000; 10: 329-41.
47. Mauro MA, Koehler RE, Baron TH. Advances in gastrointestinal intervention: the treatment of gastroduodenal and colorectal obstructions with metallic stents. *Radiology* 2000; 216: 659-69.
48. Lo SK. Metallic stenting for colorectal obstruction. *Gastrointest Endosc Clin North Am* 1999; 9: 459-73.
49. Adamsen S, Meisner S. Expandable metal stents for malignant colorectal obstruction. Techniques. *Gastrointest Endosc* 2001; 3: 103-7.

50. Baron TH. The use of self-expanding metal stents within the gastrointestinal tract. *N Engl J Med* 2001; in press.
51. Gevers AM, Macken E, Hiele M, Rutgeerts P. A comparison of laser therapy, plastic stents, and expandable metal stents for palliation of malignant dysphagia in patients without a fistula. *Gastrointest Endosc* 1998; 48: 383-8.

Management of gastrointestinal lesions with malignant potential endoscopic techniques for palliation: laser techniques

Hugh Barr

Cranfield Postgraduate Medical School in Gloucestershire, Gloucestershire Royal Hospital, Gloucester, UK

Tumour obstructing the lumen of the gastrointestinal tract can be directly targeted and destroyed by various endoscopic methods. These methods are predominantly used for the palliation of symptomatic cancer. Laser ablation using thermal or photodynamic therapy has been widely accepted and adopted and is very useful. Although, not addressed in detail in this paper, laser techniques are also very useful for the destruction of early and pre-neoplastic lesions in a minimally invasive fashion under sedation on an outpatient basis.

Laser photo thermal therapy

Absorption of a photon of light in a non-specific manner may produce thermal changes in tissue. These at present are the most widely used and surgically useful biological effects produced by a laser beam. If the rate of delivery of the photons (laser power) is such that the energy is dissipated in the surrounding medium as quickly as it is delivered no significant rise in temperature will occur. However, if the light is delivered, at high enough power, the tissue temperature will rise, and is exponentially dependent on the laser power. The thermal properties of the tissue treated are governed by three mechanisms: the ability of the tissue to transport heat by thermal conduction and diffusion, the ability to store heart and the ability to transport heat through the vascular system. Local heating of neoplastic tissue to 41-45 °C may produce selective hyperthermic damage. This differential cell kill is lost above 45 °C and all cells are rapidly destroyed above 50 °C. Further heating of the tissue causes thermal contraction and coagulation of proteins, arresting haemorrhage. If more heating occurs, necrosis is followed by vaporisation of the tissue above 100 °C.

Laser photo thermal therapy was first exploited using the Neodymium yttrium aluminium garnet (Nd: YAG) laser for the re-canalisation of obstructing oesophageal cancer in five patients in the early 1980's [1]. The laser was coupled to an optical fibre, which was passed through the instrumentation channel of the endoscope, and held approximately 0.5 cm from the tumour and used to coagulate and vaporise the obstructing lesion. An alternative technique is to use the laser in contact with the tissue with the laser beam transmitted through an artificial sapphire probe. Comparison of the techniques has shown that they are complimentary; the non-contact method is best for exophytic tumour nodules and contact therapy very useful when there is complete luminal obstruction [2].

Laser photodynamic therapy

This is method of non-thermal local tissue and tumour destruction. Cytotoxic species, predominantly singlet oxygen, are generated following the administration of a photosensitiser, and locally activated by light of appropriate wavelength. The light is usually delivered from a laser. The most commonly used method of photodynamic therapy is to administer a photosensitiser intravenously and allow retention in the tissue for 48 hours prior to irradiation with appropriate wavelength light. The discovery that an administered substance could cause photosensitivity is attributed to Oscar Raab and Professor von Tappeiner. They examined many photosensitising substances and called the phenomenon "photodynamic action/photodynamische Erscheinung". They demonstrated that a photosensitiser, light and molecular oxygen were necessary [3]. The widespread use of endoscopy allowed physicians to exploit the potential of photodynamic therapy for the palliation of gastrointestinal cancers. Large obstructing oesophageal cancers were treated with photodynamic therapy with good relief of dysphagia and possible prolongation of survival [4].

The problem of targeting the photosensitiser to the mucosa, and avoiding systemic photosensitisation may be overcome by administering a prodrug and generating the photosensitiser within the cells. The metabolic activities of the mucosal cells, which have a rapid turnover, generate the photosensitiser to a greater degree than the surrounding tissues. The generated photosensitiser tends to stay within the cells in whose mitochondria it was synthesised [5, 6]. The most widely used method involves the excess administration of 5-aminolaevulinic acid (5-ALA), with intracellular accumulation of the photosensitiser protoporphyrin IX (PpIX). The synthesis of 5-ALA from glycine and succinyl-CoA is the first step in porphyrin biosynthesis and ultimately haemoglobin. This pathway is tightly regulated by end product inhibition. If excess 5-ALA is administered, then this regulation is bypassed and an intracellular accumulation of the photosensitiser protoporphyrin IX (PpIX) is induced. The level of photosensitisation is minimised to a few hours and the 5-ALA can be administered orally. The photosensitiser is activated in tissue using 633-635 nm light from a dye laser [7].

The photo physics of photodynamic therapy are important for a full exploitation of the technique. Both administered and generated photosensitisers have specific action spectra, which are the wavelengths of light that are absorbed to produce an excited electronic state. In this state the molecule has a higher energy and is very reactive. Direct interaction with oxygen results in the generation of highly reactive cytotoxic singlet oxygen. This molecule destroys membranes by peroxidation and cells rapidly die. However, a certain concentration (threshold concentration) of the toxic photoproduct is required, and the photosensitiser is consumed by photodegradation in the process. Several photosensitisers are retained in tumours longer than in their surrounding normal tissues. At certain times after administration there exists a concentration differential of 2-3:1 between the neoplastic tissue and adjacent normal structures. Selective tumour destruction can be achieved if the photosensitiser is administered in low dosage, since the photosensitiser is photodegraded by light irradiation before the threshold photodynamic dose is reached. However, tumours that selectively retain a higher concentration of photosensitiser are destroyed because a threshold photodynamic dose is achieved and cell death occurs [8]. This selective effect is restricted to very low dose and is rarely clinically useful.

Palliation of oesophageal and gastric cancer

Obstructing oesophageal cancer can be treated on an outpatient basis with endoscopic photo thermal laser therapy. Patients tolerate treatment under sedation and the most widely used laser is the Nd: YAG, which is set to deliver 60-90 watts for 1 second pulses, and the fibre tip is kept clear of debris by a co-axially flowing gas jet. A survey of 1,359 patients treated using the laser showed that the retrograde method (therapy starting at the distal margin and working upwards) of treatment following preliminary dilatation of the oesophagus was most widely used [9]. Prograde treatment (starting at the upper surface of the tumour) requires more experience and carries an increased risk of perforation. However, it may be required in patients with total obstruction. Complications occur in approximately 5% with an overall procedure related mortality of 1%. The commonest complication is oesophageal perforation (2.5%), followed by fistulation (1%), haemorrhage (0.75%) and sepsis (0.5%). Many of the perforations are related to the preliminary dilatation rather than the subsequent laser treatment [10]. Laser therapy allowed most patients to achieve a near normal diet immediately after treatment but recurrent dysphagia is a major problem *(Table I)*.

Table I. The quality of swallowing after endoscopic laser therapy

Patients Total number	Mortality (%)	Normal diet (%)	Soft diet (%)	Liquid diet (%)	Recurrent dysphagia (%)	Reference
18	0	38	28	22	22	[11]
62	1.6	81	13	7	60	[9]
28	0	92	8		29	[12]
34	3	74	21	5	53	[13]
76	3	86	86	10	11	[10]
86	2	67	12		65	[14]

Thus, most patients will require repeated treatments, and most centres space treatment at 4-6 weekly intervals. Strategies to prevent recurrent dysphagia and prolong the dysphagia free interval have involved combination therapy with external beam or intraluminal radiotherapy. The dysphagia free interval was prolonged [15], but fibrous stricture proved to be a major problem (30%). Some patients had prolonged survival with minimal endoscopic intervention [16]. The addition of external beam radiotherapy with palliative laser recannalisation of the tumour allowed 70% of patients to be palliated until death a mean of 6 months later [17].

There are now several non-laser methods for palliation of obstructing oesophageal cancer. It is clear that self-expanding stents are safer than the rigid prostheses [18], and may be associated with longer dysphagia free interval with greater improvement in dysphagia score. However there were more complications than following endoscopic laser therapy [19]. Our randomised study comparing self-expanding metal prostheses with endoscopic laser therapy demonstrated no difference in efficacy of uncovered self-expanding metal prostheses and the laser for the palliation of oesophageal cancer *(Table II)*.

Table II. A randomised comparison of endoscopic laser therapy with self-expanding metal stent insertion for the palliation of malignant dysphagia

	Self-expanding prosthesis uncovered (9 patients)	Endoscopic laser therapy (12 patients)
Dysphagia grade (0-9 scale). Mean pre-treatment	3	3
Dysphagia grade (0-9 scale). Mean post-treatment	6	6
Stricture size (mm). Pre-treatment	5	5
Stricture size (mm). Mean post-treatment	10	10
Weight (kg). Pre-treatment	60	61
Weight (kg). Mean post-treatment	59	60
Mean survival (weeks)	17	15

Laser and other thermal methods of tumour destruction have similar effects, whether an expensive laser or a cheaper device such as an Argon-Plasma coagulator (APC) is used. Tissue can be vaporized and coagulated either to remove obstruction or arrest bleeding. The APC is generally felt to be less efficient than laser coagulation and more treatments may be required to produce the desired effect [20]. Thermal laser therapy can on occasion be effective in arresting or decreasing hemorrhage from large bleeding gastric cancers. The technique must be altered from superficial surface laser ablation to interstitial contact laser therapy to coagulate the central bulk of the cancer. The laser is inserted into the tumour and a lower power is used over a longer period to coagulate the tumour. This has been shown to reduce the transfusion requirements of patients with advanced inoperable bleeding gastric cancer [21].

A large randomized comparison (236 patients) of thermal laser with photodynamic therapy (PDT) showed that both were equally effective for the palliation of malignant dysphagia. PDT was associated with temporary photosensitivity but was easier to perform and associated with fewer perforations (PDT-1%, thermal laser-7%) [22]. Photodynamic therapy may be particularly useful for patients with very long tortuous tumours, blocked stents and high tumours. Injection of alcohol and intra-tumoral chemotherapy can also be very useful. As with PDT and thermal therapy treatment often has to be repeated. These methods may be particularly useful if there is tumour in-growth or overgrowth of a prosthesis [23]. Some large series have demonstrated quite prolonged survival in patients treated with thermal laser therapy with a 4% of 211 patients surviving 2 years. There seemed to little survival improvement with the addition of adjuvant chemotherapy or radiotherapy [24].

Photodynamic therapy is proving particularly useful for pre-cancerous and early cancers. If the patient is frail or with concomitant disease, and unlikely to tolerate more radical therapy, then photodynamic therapy may be highly effective and give prolonged disease control and prevent progression to metastatic cancer [25-27]. Combination therapy with radiotherapy and chemotherapy seems to add little survival benefit to the effect of photodynamic therapy alone [28]. Recently, combination therapy with hyperbaric oxygenation has appeared to enhance the effect of photodynamic therapy [29], but possibly at the price of increasing the incidence of tracheo-oesophageal fistula in patients with T4 cancers when compared to other series [30].

Palliation of duodenal and ampullary cancer

Both photodynamic therapy and laser photo thermal therapy have been used to treat ampullary, peri-ampullary and duodenal cancer [31]. It can produce prolonged survival and has the potential to prevent duodenal obstruction and obviate the need for duodenal stenting procedures. There is little data on the overall effects of laser therapy. For the treatment of ampullary tumours the bile duct must be stented prior to laser therapy. If this is not done, then fibrosis of the outlet inevitably leads to further jaundice. *Table III* shows the two series that have been reported.

Table III. Outcomes of photo thermal laser therapy for ampullary and duodenal tumours

	Complications	Recurrent jaundice (%)	Duodenal obstruction (%)	Mean survival months
Fowler *et al.*, 1999 [31]. 12 patients	0	17	8	20
Lambert *et al.* 1988 [32]. 8 patients	12	24	19	6

Palliation of colorectal cancer

Most patients with colon and rectal cancer are palliated using surgical techniques. However, endoscopic laser therapy is very effective at destroying large areas tumour, relieving the dreadful symptoms of tenesmus, abnormal discharge, obstruction and bleeding. Pain associated with local invasion is poorly controlled, as are the symptoms of incontinence associated with rectal cancer locally invasive into the sphincters [33]. There are other techniques that can be used to debulk and palliate advancing inoperable rectal cancer, most notable endoscopic transanal resection (ETAR) using the urological resectoscope. This latter technique often has to be performed under general or regional anaesthesia. A comparison of symptom control has shown that ETAR was more effective in controlling the symptoms. The technique was also often completed at one session whereas laser therapy required repeated treatments to keep the tumour under control *(Table IV)*. However, ETAR carried a greater morbidity and mortality [34].

Table IV. Comparison of endoscopic laser therapy with endoscopic transanal resection for the palliation of rectal cancer

	Rectal bleeding abolished (%)	Abnormal discharge (%)	Tenesmus abolished (%)	30 day mortality (%)	Morbidity (%)
Endoscopic laser therapy. 65 patients	31	30	17	3	1.5
Endoscopic transanal resection. 41 patients	65	63	75	10	12

Conclusions

Endoscopic palliation using the laser is a very important and useful technique, but must be regarded as complimentary to other methods.

References

1. Fleischer D, Kessler F, Haye D. Endoscopic Nd YAG laser therapy for carcinoma of the esophagus: a new palliative approach. *Am J Surg* 1982; 143: 280-3.
2. Ell Ch. Hochberger J, Lux G. Clinical experience of non-contact and contact Nd:YAG laser therapy for inoperable malignant stenoses of the esophagus and stomach. *Lasers Med Sci* 1986; 1: 143-6.
3. Tappeiner von H. Die photodynamische erscheinung. *Ergebnisse der Physiologie* 1999; 8: 698-741.
4. McCaughen JS, Hicks W, Laufman L, May E, Roach R. Palliation of esophageal malignancy with photoradiation therapy. *Cancer* 1984; 54: 2905-10.
5. Gray MW, Burger G, Lang BF. Mitochondral evolution. *Science* 1999; 283: 1476-81.
6. Kennedy JC, Pottier RH. Endogenous protoporphyrin, a clinically useful photosensitiser for photodynamic therapy. *J Photochem Photobiol* 1992; 14: 275-84.

7. Barr H, Dix AJ, Kendall C, Stone N. The potential for photodynamic therapy in the management of upper gastrointestinal disease alimentary. *Pharmacol Ther* 2001; 15: 311-21.
8. Barr H, Tralau CJ, Boulos PB, Krasner N, Clark CG, Bown SG. Selective destruction of dimethylhydrazine rat colon cancer using phothalocyanine photodynamic therapy. *Gastroenterology* 1990; 98: 1532-7.
9. Ell Ch, Reimann RF, Lux G, Demling L. Palliative laser treatment of malignant stenoses in the upper gastrointestinal tract. *Endoscopy* 1986; 18: 21-6.
10. Krasner N, Barr H, Skidmore C, Morris I Palliative laser therapy for malignant dysphagia. *Gut* 1987; 28: 792-8.
11. Moon BC, Woolfson IK, Mercer CD. Neodymiumyttrium aluminium garnet laser vaporization for palliation of esophageal carcinoma. *J Thor Cardiovasc Surg* 1989; 98: 11-4.
12. Buset M, des Marez B, Batze M, Bourgeois N, de Boelpaepe C, de Tœuf J, Cremer M. Palliative endoscopic management of obstructive oesophageal cancer: laser or prosthesis? *Gastrointest Endosc* 1989; 33: 357-61.
13. Bown SG, Hawes R, Matthewson K, Swain CP, Barr H, Boulos PB, Clark CG. Endoscopic laser palliation for advanced malignant dysphagia. *Gut* 1987; 28: 799-807.
14. Shumeli E, Myszor MF, Burke D, Record CO, Mathewson K. Limitation of laser treatment for malignant dysphagia. *Br J Surg* 1992; 79: 778-80.
15. Spencer GM, Thorpe SM, Sargent IR, Blackman GM, Solano J, Tobias JS, Bown SG. Laser and brachytherapy in palliation of adencarcinoma of the oesophagus and cardia. *Gut* 1996; 39: 726-31.
16. Shumeli E, Srivastava E, Dawes JDH, Claque M, Mathewson K, Record CO. Combination of laser treatment and intraluminal radiotherapy for malignant dysphagia. *Gut* 1996; 38: 803-5.
17. Bourke MJ, Hope RL, Chu G, Gillespie PE, Bull C, O'Rourke I, Williams SJ. Laser palliation of inoperable malignant dysphagia initial and at death. *Gastrointest Endosc* 1996; 43: 29-32.
18. Knyrium K, Wagner HJ, Bethge N, Kemling M, Vakil N. A controlled trial of an expansile stent for palliation of esophageal obstruction due to inoperable cancer. *N Engl J Med* 1993; 329: 1302-07.
19. Saunders M, Tan B, Ellul J, Watkinson A, Adam A, Mason R. Prospective triple randomised trial of laser *vs* expandable metal (covered and uncovered) stents in the management of inoperable oesophageal carcinoma-preliminary results. *Gut* 1995; 37: A4.
20. Gossner L, Ell C. Malignant stricture thermal treatment. *Gastrointest Endosc Clin North Am* 1998; 8: 493-501.
21. Barr H, Krasner N. Intestinal laser photocoagulation for treating bleeding gastric cancer. *Br Med J* 1989; 299: 659-60.
22. Lightdale CJ, Heier SK, Marcon NE, *et al.* Photodynamic therapy with porfimer sodium *versus* thermal ablation therapy with Nd:YAG laser for palliation of esophageal cancer: a multicentre randomized trial. *Gastrointest Endosc* 1995; 42: 507-12.
23. Saidi RF, Marcon NE. Non-thermal ablation of malignant esophageal stricture. *Gastrointest Endosc Clin North Am* 1998; 8: 465-91.
24. Savage AP, Baigrie RJ, Cobb RA, Barr H, Kettlewell MGW. Palliation of malignant dysphagia by laser therapy. *Dis Esoph* 1997; 10: 243-6.
25. Barr H. Photodynamic therapy in Gastrointestinal Cancer: a realistic option? *Drugs Aging* 2000; 16: 81-6.
26. Barr H, Shepherd NA, Dix A, Roberts DJH, Tan WC, Krasner N. Eradication of high grade dysplasia in columnar-lined (Barrett's) oesophagus using photodynamic therapy with endogenously generated protoporphyrin IX. *Lancet* 1996; 348: 584-5.
27. Overholt BF, Panjepour M, Haydek JM. Photodynamic therapy for Barrett's esophagus: follow-up in 100 patients. *Gastrointest Endosc* 1999; 49: 1-7.
28. Sibille A, Lambert R, Souquet JC, Sabben G, Descos F. Long-term survival after photodynamic therapy for esophageal cancer. *Gastroenterology* 1995; 108: 337-44.

29. Maier A, Tomaselli F, Anegg U, Fehak P, Fell B, Luznik S, Pinter H, Smolle-Juttner FM. Combined photodynamic therapy and hyperbaric oxygenation in carcinoma of the esophagus and the esophago-gastric junction. *Eur J Cardiothorac Surg* 2000; 18; 649-55.
30. Moghissi K, Dixon K, Thorpe JAC, Stringer M, Moore PJ. The role of photodynamic therapy in inoperable oesophageal cancer. *Eur J Cardiothorac Surg* 2000; 17: 95-100.
31. Fowler A, Barham PB, Britton BJ, Barr H. Laser ablation of ampullary cancer. *Endoscopy* 1999: 31; 745-7.
32. Lambert R, Ponchon T, Chavaillon A, Berger F. Laser treatment of tumours of the papilla of Vater. *Endoscopy* 1988; 20: 227-31.
33. McGown I, Barr H, Krasner N. Palliative laser therapy for inoperable rectal cancer-does it work? A prospective study of quality of life. *Cancer* 1989; 63: 967-9.
34. Barr H. Laser phototherapy for gastrointestinal neoplasia. University of Liverpool ChM thesis, 1995: 161-9.

Achevé d'imprimer par Corlet, Imprimeur, S.A.
14110 Condé-sur-Noireau (France)
N° d'Imprimeur : 54411 - Dépôt légal : septembre 2001

Imprimé en U.E.